D1622019

The Campitelli Advanced Method for a Flat Abdomen and Thin Waist

by Frank Campitelli and Chef Edward Valente

Copyright ©1995 by The Hanford Press

All rights reserved. No part of this publication book may be reproduced,
stored in a retrieval system, or transmitted, in any form or by any
means, electronic, mechanical, photocopying, recording or otherwise
without the prior written permission of the publisher.

Printed in the United States of America.
Published simultaneously in Canada.

IMPORTANT HEALTH INFORMATION

The information contained in this book is intended to help you make informed decisions about your diet and health, not to substitute for any treatment that may have been prescribed by your physician. If you suspect that you have a medical problem, we urge you to seek competent medical help. Keep in mind that nutritional needs vary from person to person, depending on age, sex, health status and total diet. Anyone considering a weight management or exercise program should obtain approval from their health care provider before beginning such a program. Because there may be some individual risk involved, the publisher and researchers are not responsible for any adverse effects or consequences resulting from the use or misuse of any of the suggestions, preparations, procedures, recipes or other content in this book.

CREDITS

Publishing Director	Robert Concoby
Production Director	Rochelle Crews
Art Director	Dan Zola
Graphic Designers	Nancy Giermann Cappy Petri
Writers	Robert Concoby David Nicol Robert Villella
Editors	Michael McNulty Louise McNulty
Photographers	David Baio Brandon Hemphill
Researchers	Flo Lynn Jack Lynn
Project Coordinator	Sherri Peters
Proofreaders	Chris Trumphour Robyn Bennington
MEDLINE Medical Researcher	Robert Concoby

A very special Thank You goes to the Akron City Club Board of Governors and Judd Limbach, Club Manager, for letting us use their extraordinary facility. We also want to thank the Akron City Club's two talented Sous Chefs, David Eichorn and Anthony Collins, for their invaluable assistance in food preparation and recipe testing. They prepared and stylized many of the gourmet meals photographed for this book.

TABLE OF CONTENTS

INTRODUCTION

Fat. The word sounds bad. And looks bad on paper. As if that isn't enough, it looks even worse when it takes up a seemingly permanent residence on our bodies, usually in places where we don't want it to reside.

Mankind has gone to unending, and sometimes ridiculous, lengths to lose weight. Most often, the results are less than satisfying.

Grapefruit diets, plastic body wraps, sauna suits, gritty, gruesome fiber drinks and magic pills by the untold millions attempt to fill the public's insatiable demand for relief from the burden of overweight.

The answer is so much simpler and less expensive than all those alternatives. Scientifically-based on human physiology, the answer's been right in front of us. What's the answer to losing weight? Simply this ...

Eat.

Then take a pleasant walk.

When you get hungry, eat some more.

The human body is well-suited to both of these activities, eating and walking. We've discovered in the last few years that eating the right foods can actually increase weight loss, while keeping us emotionally happy as well. And a daily walk boosts the metabolism quite nicely.

A fringe benefit of eating right and exercising is a fit and trim body that works well, both on the outside and the inside. Lowered blood pressure and a decreased risk of cancer or heart disease have been proven to accompany a low-fat eating plan and some form of moderate exercise.

Chef Edward Valente of the Akron City Club has developed wonderfully simple and delicious gourmet meals that help you lose weight the low-fat way. He has lost 65 pounds himself following this very plan.

Certified Trainer Frank Campitelli designs customized exercise plans for his clients that super-power weight loss and accelerate muscle gain. A 14-year weight training veteran, he has helped countless dozens of people become fit and trim in only minutes a day.

These two men have now joined forces to produce what is unquestionably the finest low-fat eating and exercise plan in the world today — The Biotech Method.

Using the very latest in nutritional and physical training technology, they will show you how to eat all the food you want and still lose weight. Or, they can show you how to achieve maximum muscle gain through a combination of proper food and exercise.

And in less than 25 minutes a day, you can exercise most every muscle in your body to its ripped maximum using Frank's exclusive exercise plan.

The journey to a fit and trim body takes only minutes a day. And you don't need to suffer through hunger pangs from calorie counting or excruciating pain from gut-wrenching physical training. That's the old way.

Join us now on the new way — the Biotech Way. It's a delightful and rewarding journey to a brand new you.

Robert Concoby

FOREWORD

As a practicing cardiovascular surgeon for 22 years, and having seen first hand the ravages of ill-health, it was a delight for me to read this very clear, informative, and enticing description of a way to avoid the need for services of people such as myself.

Anyone in the healthcare field would have to be aware that the quality of life in our highly-developed western civilization seems to be less than what it could be with what we now know of modern science. As much as I have labored in the operating room, hundreds, if not thousands, of researchers have labored both in laboratories and at computers for years trying to analyze causes of disease. Through many epidemicalogical studies of people with different lifestyles, it has been shown that there definitely is an influence from one's activities. In this book, the authors document many of the detailed studies that are virtually universally accepted to be of relevance to one degree or another, and show that when it is all put together these can definitely influence one's chances of not only living longer but living better.

For many years I have personally observed some (but unfortunately not enough) of the suggestions brought out here and have, to a much lesser degree, followed the literature on prevention and lifestyle influences. I was pleasantly surprised to learn a great deal from this material that even I was not current with. The extensive documentation certainly is commendable and is available to anyone who might want to look up the basic references themselves. I think it is safe to say that no one can gainsay the observations made here and it is up to us as individuals to put these good practices into effect. In addition to the documentation of the scientific basis, Chef Valente has shown many delightful ways of implementing this particularly in regard to eating better. It behooves us all to select "al a carte" from this informative menu as to whether we choose to take more vitamins or eat more greens or both, but in any case we have a very thorough presentation of the scientific validity of same. Though the results do not always become apparent within a matter of days or weeks, I am totally convinced that they do so over a period of time.

Needless to say, all of the following insights will be of benefit but obviously the greatest benefit will come from the greater application of the greater number of these including the dietary supplements, exercise regimens, and most importantly, more healthy eating habits.

Dr. David M. Sokol, M.D.

Part One

How To
Flatten Abdominal Bulge
By Eliminating
The Four Main Causes

THE FIVE CAUSES OF LOWER ABDOMINAL BULGE

Excess abdominal fat raises our risk of various diseases, among them heart disease, high cholesterol, high blood pressure and diabetes.

Our experience shows that both men and women tend to get thicker around the middle as they grow older. Sadly, fellows, we men tend to have more of a problem with "potbellies" than do women.

In this chapter, we'll discuss the reasons that we grow fat around our middle. Then we'll detail some very simple but effective ways to slow down and even eliminate the abdominal fat-gaining process.

WHY WE HAVE BIG STOMACHS

Many of the causes of excess abdominal fat are lifestyle and occupation-related. While some of the causes are beyond our control, we can always adjust our lifestyles and respond properly to those causes. As a result, we can be healthier, and fit and trim.

POOR POSTURE

By far, the biggest reason for bulging abdomens is poor posture and weakened supporting muscles in the belly, back and shoulders.

This can be seen in what we call torso drooping and slumped shoulders. These are both caused by a lack of muscle tone and strength in the trapezius, rhomboids, lats, and rear deltoid muscles. These muscle groups help pull the shoulders back. If they are weak and the shoulders aren't pulled back sufficiently, the shoulders then droop forward.

Along with this, the head, neck and chin fall down, pulling the dereistic area of the vertebrae into a heavy curvature. All of this combines to push the rib cage and diaphragm down, which makes the stomach protrude. Fortunately, all of these problems can be solved using simple strengthening techniques.

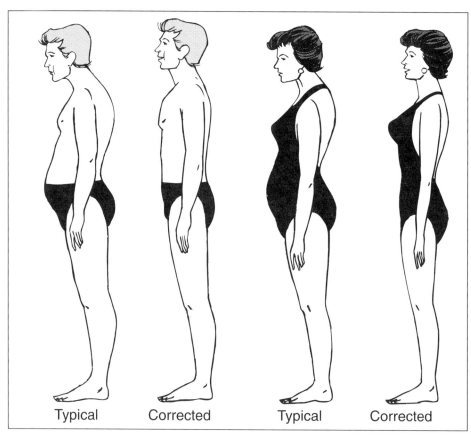

| Typical | Corrected | Typical | Corrected |

Another cause of lower abdominal bulge is actually weak muscles in other areas of the body which cause bad posture and misalignment of body parts. Excess fat is also one of the causes of lower abdominal bulge but more so for men than for women. The main fat storage area for men is the abdomen but the main fat storage area for women is the hips and thighs. Typical male and female profiles are to the left and the corrected profiles using the Campitelli Advanced Method are to the right.

Have you ever seen somebody standing and pulling and sucking in a big breath of air, their chest comes up and their stomach goes in. You can achieve this look almost subconsciously when the proper muscle groups are strong, and also stretched in the right places.

Certain occupations demand particular postures which many times inadvertently lead to excess abdominal fat. For many people, jobs which require them to remain seated throughout the day contribute to a larger stomach. For others, some jobs demand that people lean over and work with their arms in front of them. Some of these varied occupations include office workers, surgeons, opticians, truck drivers and the like.

Other occupations require people to stand, yet still work with their arms unsupported and away from their body, such as hairdressers, barbers, construction workers and factory assembly-line jobs.

All these occupations have one thing in common: they require the workers to have their arms out in front of them, and to put a lot of weight on the upper back and shoulders. This causes poor posture, makes the shoulders droop, and pushes the rib cage and diaphragm down. All of the belly-busting problems associated with these occupational stresses can be corrected with stretching and strengthening of the appropriate muscle groups.

IMPROPER BREATHING

Astonishingly, poor breathing is a contributor to poor health for many people today.

Many modern ailments such as back pain, headache, depression, moodiness, high blood pressure and other stress-related illnesses can have their beginnings in improper breathing.

We shall examine in-depth the peer-review study done by Dr. Shealy at his Shealy Institute documenting the many benefits of their process called gravity-centered breathing.

PREGNANCY

For women, a big contributor to a protruding abdomen is the after-effects of pregnancy. Being pregnant stretches the abdominal wall due to the baby being right under the abdominal muscle groups. This also adds a lot of weight in the front part of the torso, sometimes up to twenty-five pounds, and even more. Pregnancy also adds muscle stress to the upper and lower back. These muscle groups tighten and cause the torso to slump.

Along with an out-of-align back slump, the pelvis also rotates forward. This makes the buttocks stick out because the back part of your pelvis is rotated up while the front part of the pelvis is pushed downwards.

Without some muscle retraining after pregnancy, the pelvic area may not fully return to its normal position. The buttocks remain overextended, and the lower abdomen is still pushed down in the front. All of these muscle groups can be retrained quite simply and easily, and return to their normal toned condition.

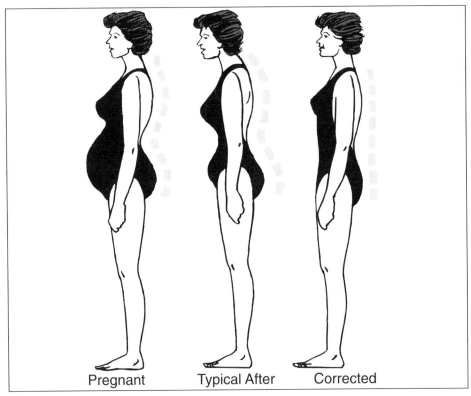

| Pregnant | Typical After | Corrected |

Childbearing is yet another cause of lower abdominal bulge but not so much from stretched skin as most people believe. The biggest cause is the fact that during pregnancy, the pelvic bone is tilted to the rear and the buttocks also extend in that direction. But after pregnancy, in most cases the pelvic area does not shift back to its normal position which causes the buttocks to remain overextended to the rear and the lower abdomen to be over extended in front. But this can be corrected with the Campitelli Advanced Method.

LOWER ABS NOT STRONG

Another abdominal problem is that the lower abdominal muscles are weak. Most of the time, these muscles deteriorate due to lack of exercise. Since most occupations do not require any type of abdominal contraction, they become weak due to the lack of stress. If stress is introduced in the form of exercises, such as crunches or abs, the problem is almost completely eliminated.

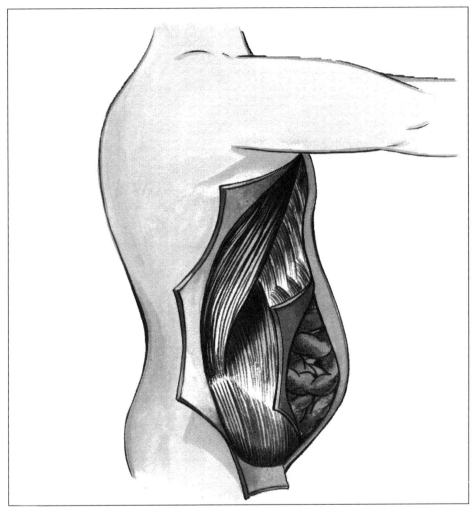

One of the causes of lower abdominal bulge is the fact that the lower abdominal wall is much thinner than the upper abdominal wall. This causes the intestines to push out the lower abdominal area much like a bubble in the weak area of a tire. This problem can be solved with the Campitelli Advanced Method.

OVERWEIGHT AND ABDOMINAL FAT

Obviously overweight or obesity plays a large role in a big belly. Basically, the weight of the upper body collapses onto the rib cage. This weight pushes the lower abdomen out. Combined with this, the additional stress placed on the upper body over-stretches the shoulders. As a result, less muscle strength is available to keep the rib cage vertical. The rib cage collapses, and this adds to push the abdomen out further.

A common problem in many people is the high percentage of interabdominal fat. Many people have large abdomen areas or torsos but have small legs. This is due to the high amount of fat that surrounds the intestines and abdominal organs to keep them from experiencing shock from physical activities.

This excess interabdominal fat is otherwise known as the "beer belly" or the "pot belly." In many instances, "pot bellies," while almost completely composed of excess fat, is very hard and actually doesn't seem to have a lot of fat on it. This is very common in men and in women with certain body types. The good news is this: pot bellies can be modified through diet, using the tips we've discussed throughout the book.

Our modern lifestyle also contributes greatly to poor abdominal tone. Abdominal muscles don't get exercised to the degree necessary in our post-Industrial Revolution workplace.

The bad news is that almost everybody has all or some of these abdominal fat problems. And many of the reasons for having a pot belly are interrelated. Some problems cause others to happen.

The GOOD news is that The Campitelli Advanced Method can solve all of these problems in only minutes a day. The remaining chapters will show you how to fix all your abdominal problems quickly and easily!

2

How To Correct Lower Abdomen Bulge Caused By Weak Abdominal Muscles

Weak abdominal muscles contribute to a "pot belly" in several different ways. The obvious result of weak abs is their inability to hold in the organs of the lower abdominal cavity — thus allowing them to "spill" out from under the rib cage and above the pubic bone. But, there are two not so obvious consequences:

(1) an improper curvature to the lower spine and

(2) a downward rotation of the pelvis.

Both of these bad posture conditions highly exaggerate a protruding belly.

To evaluate your posture and, specifically, to determine the presence of a sway back or tilted pelvis, see chapter 6.

Five different muscle groups control bending and twisting of the lower trunk and work to hold in the contents of the middle and lower abdomen. Understanding the anatomy and physiology of these muscle groups will help determine the major reasons for a protruding pooch and also suggest a specific course of action for correcting the problem.

Three flat muscles and a band-shaped muscle form the front and sides of the abdominal basket and one 4-sided muscle forms the back. The muscles of the front and sides of the abdominal wall are arranged in three layers, with the fibers in each layer running in different directions much like the layers of wood in a sheet of plywood. The result is a very strong "girdle" of muscle that covers and supports the abdominal cavity and its internal organs.

The three layers in the side of the abdominal wall are arranged as follows, going from the outside of the body toward the spine:

Outer Layer — External Obliques

Middle Layer — Internal Obliques

Inner Layer — Transversus Abdominus

These three groups of flat muscles work together to twist the trunk and to bend the trunk at the waist. They are also active as a unit with the rectus abdominus during breathing and functions that require increased intra-abdominal pressure — such as straining, defecation, forced expiration and childbirth.

In addition to these sheet-like muscles, the band-shaped muscle — rectus abdominus — runs down the midline of the abdomen from under the breast bone to the pubic bone. Although the other muscles have physiological importance, the rectus abdominus and the external obliques are the primary muscles that we can see since they are so close to the skin's surface.

RECTUS ABDOMINUS

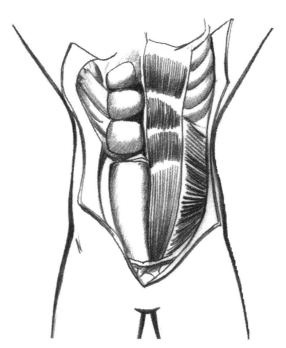

The rectus abdominus compresses the abdomen and pulls the front of the pelvis upward, thereby flattening the lumbar curve of the spine. Plus it compresses the abdominal cavity, aiding in straining, defecation, forced expiration, childbirth, etc., as well as flexing the trunk.

This long shield-shaped muscle is the primary vertical muscle of the front abdominal wall. It is three times as wide at the top as it is at the bottom. The rectus abdominus is wrapped in a sheath — like a glove — that is formed by the tendonous extensions of the obliques and the transversus abdominus.

Starting from the pubic bone and pubic crest in the central region of the pelvis, the rectus abdominus runs straight up the middle of the belly and connects onto a small triangular bone attached to the lowest part of the breast bone and the cartilage between the 5th to 7th ribs. It is separated vertically in the middle by the linea alba that is a tendonous sheet with a width between a half and one inch. This tendon stretches from the breast bone to the center of the pubic bone. As a result, the abdominal wall appears to have a left and right half to it.

The front layer of the rectus sheath is firmly attached to the rectus muscle at three tendonous intersections. These tendonous intersections create the grooves in the rectus muscle and cause the muscle fiber to bulge in sections when it is tensed.

When both right and left halves of this muscle contract, the upper trunk is pulled forward. When only contracting on the left side, the trunk is pulled sideways toward the left side of the body. Likewise, contraction on only the right side of the rectus abdominus will cause the trunk to be pulled to the right.

The following exercise will strengthen this muscle.

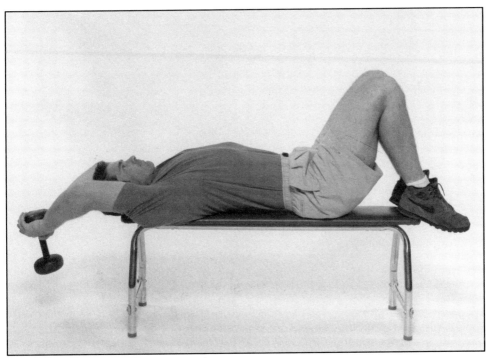

Dumbell pullover exercise movement.

EXTERNAL OBLIQUES

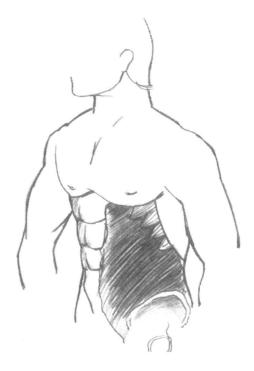

External obliques are the largest of the three flat abdominal muscles and, as we have already learned, they are the closest to the skin's surface. They lie on each side of the torso and they compress the abdomen, pull the front of the pelvis upward and thereby flatten the lumbar curve of the spine, help stabilize the torso, and twist it from side to side.

The top end of the external obliques are anchored to seven different ribs — 5 through 12 – and the bottom ends are attached to the pubic bone, the iliac bone of the pelvis and also a structure called the linea alba. The muscle fibers run from the side toward the center of the abdomen in the same direction that your fingers would point, if you were to put your hands in your pockets. As it moves toward the center it forms a flat fan-shaped muscle.

As these muscles contract, they rock the pelvis forward toward the rib cage. When the right external oblique contracts alone, the trunk and shoulders twist to the left. Conversely, when the left external oblique contracts alone, the trunk and shoulders twist to the right. And, when they contract simultaneously, the body bends at the waist drawing the head toward the feet. Obliques that are out of tone tend to sag when at rest allowing the organs of the lower abdomen to create the infamous bulge.

INTERNAL OBLIQUES

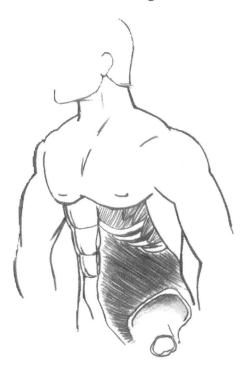

Like the external obliques, the internal obliques lie on each side of the torso and they compress the abdomen. They also pull the front of the pelvis upward and thereby flatten the lumbar curve of the spine, help stabilize the torso, and twist it from side to side.

Internal obliques are sandwiched by the two other flat abdominal muscles, the external obliques and the transversus abdominus, and therefore are not visible. The bottom ends of the internal obliques are anchored in a thick connective tissue sheath located in the lower back — called the thoracolumbar facia — and also from a region of the prominent bones of the hip, the iliac bone. The fibers run at right angles to the external oblique muscle. They fan out from their anchor points running diagonally upward in approximately the direction that your thumb points when you place your four fingers in your front pants pockets with your thumb opened as far as it will go.

The top ends of the internal obliques connect to the lowest three or four ribs, where they become continuous with the respiratory muscles of the rib cage — the internal intercostal muscles. As these muscles simultaneously contract, they pull the upper trunk forward toward the feet. In contrast to the function of the external oblique, the internal oblique will twist the body towards the right if only the right side contracts, and toward the left if only the left side of the muscle contracts.

TRANSVERSUS ABDOMINUS

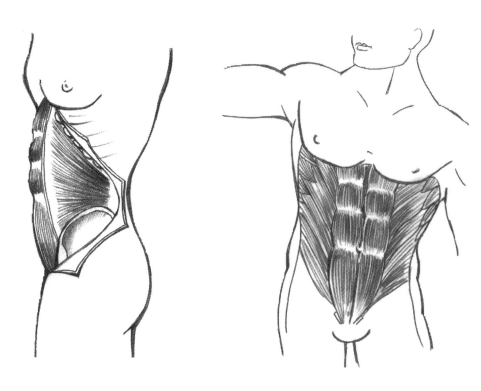

     The transversus abdominus muscles are the innermost of the three flat abdominal muscle groups. In shape and function, they resemble a girdle. The end fibers are anchored in back and then travel around the sides, straight across the tummy and connect to the linea alba and the center of the pubic bone in the front. These muscles aid in twisting and bending but do their most effective work during an attempt to draw the stomach inward.

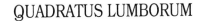

QUADRATUS LUMBORUM

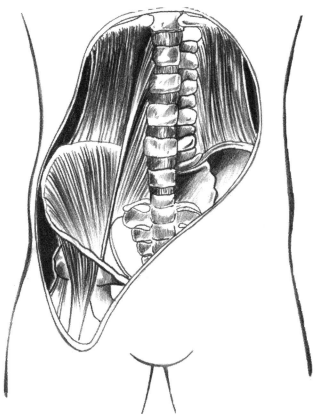

The quadratus lumborum is a thick four-sided muscle. It begins from the iliac bones of the hip and the lower lumbar vertebrae. It narrows from a rather broad base as it ascends to its connection point which is just behind the diaphragm on the 12th lowest rib and the upper lumbar vertebrae. This is a deep muscle and therefore it cannot be seen. Nevertheless, it is very active and important. If it contracts on only one side at a time, it can bend the trunk toward the same side that is contracting

When this muscle is strong and developed it is able to keep the pelvis level and therefore, it will maintain a good posture line in the lower back. It is also important in preventing the lower portion of a lateral "s" curvature of the vertebral column (scoliosis).

The following exercises will strengthen all of these muscle groups.

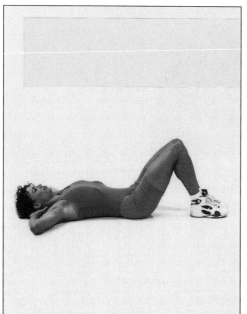

Crunch (begin)

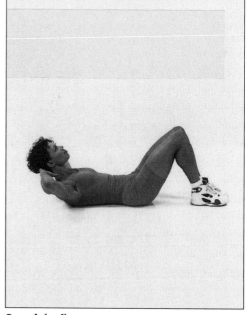

Crunch (end)

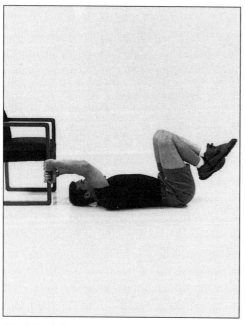

Tuck (begin)

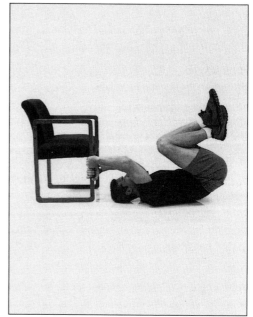

Tuck (end)

AB TRAINING TIPS

If you determine that the major problem with an unsightly bulge at your girth is the weakness of your abdominal muscles, here are some tips that will help you to strengthen and return tone to your natural muscular girdle.

1) Concentrate on exercises, in which the rib cage and pelvis are squeezed together, rather than on exercises that require a lot of hip movement.

2) Abdominal muscles can be worked more frequently than other muscles without over training, so two or three short sessions a day can yield quicker results than one long daily workout.

3) The number of repetitions you do in a set for abs depends on how hard you "crunch" at the top of each movement. Unless your abs are already extremely tired, you should probably do about 15 repetitions, but if you can do more than 25 or 30, you're probably not getting enough intensity in each repetition.

4) Working your abdominals at the end of a session can help improve the efficiency of these exercises.

3

How To Correct Your Abdomen Bulge Caused By Poor Posture

By far, one of the biggest reasons for bulging abdomens is poor posture and weakened supporting muscles in the belly, back and shoulders.

Anything that makes the spine curve too much can make your stomach look larger. Simply stated, long spines lead to flatter stomachs, while shorter spines make our tummies stick out. Big tummies are almost always accompanied by poor posture and shortened spines. Fortunately, as we'll see later, we can all do some basic things to help "elongate" our spines.

Poor posture can most easily be seen in what we call torso drooping and slumped shoulders. These are both caused by a lack of muscle tone and strength in the trapezius, rhomboids, lats, and rear deltoid muscles. These muscle groups help pull the shoulders back. If they are weak and the shoulders aren't pulled back sufficiently, the shoulders then droop forward.

Along with this, the head, neck and chin fall down, pulling the dereistic area of the vertebrae into a heavy curvature. All of this combines to push the rib cage and diaphragm down, which makes the stomach protrude. Fortunately, all these problems can be solved using simple strengthening techniques.

Have you ever seen somebody standing and pulling and sucking in a big breath of air, their chest comes up and their stomach goes in. You can achieve this look almost subconsciously when the proper muscle groups are strong, and also stretched in the right places.

The following exercises will strengthen the various muscle groups needed for good posture.

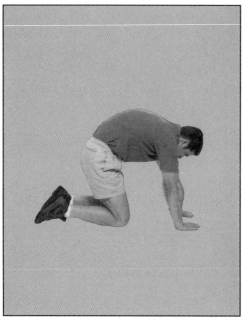

Kneeling Back Arch for stretching erector spinae (low back)

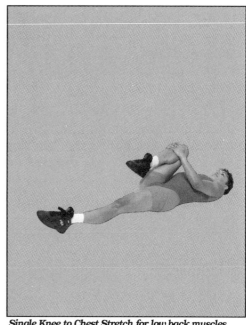

Single Knee to Chest Stretch for low back muscles

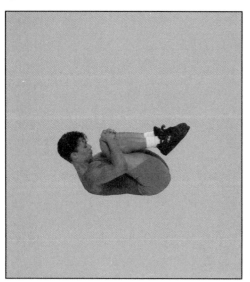

Double Knee to Chest Stretch (same muscle groups as Single Knee Stretch)

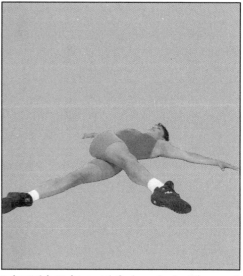

Lying Pelvic Twist stretch for lower back, obliques and gluteus maximus

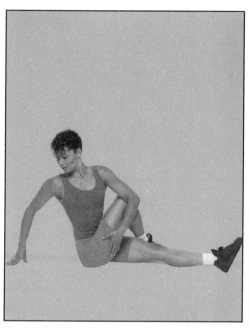

Seated Pelvic Twist for lower back, obliques and gluteus maximus

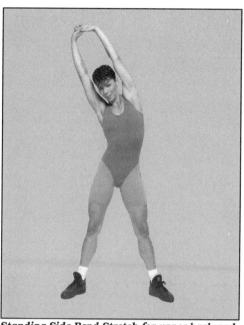

Standing Side Bend Stretch for upper back and rib cage, latissimus dorsi, intercostals and serratus anterior

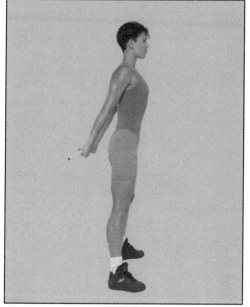

Rear Shoulder Stretch for anterior and medial deltoids and pectoral major

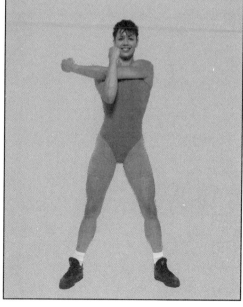

Front Shoulder Stretch for upper back trapezius, rhomboids and posterior deltoid

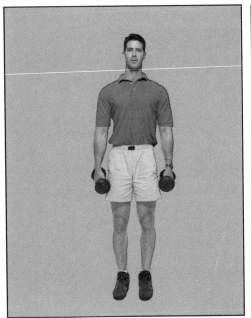
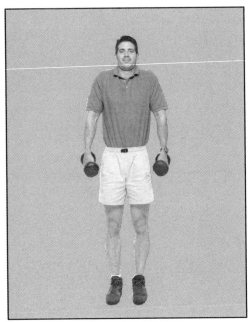

Dumbell Shrug exercise movement for trapezius muscle

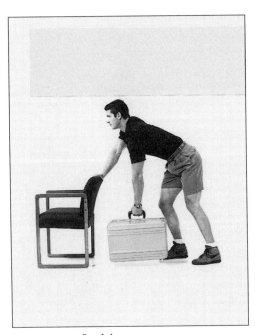
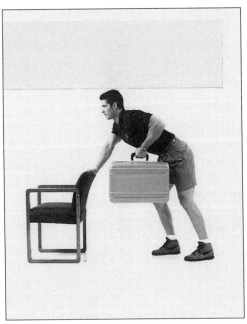

One arm row (begin)

One arm row (end)
(Switch and do with other arm also.)

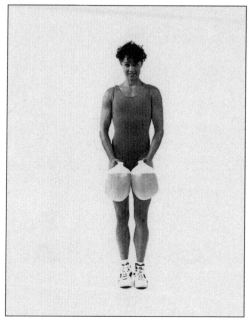

Upright Row (begin)

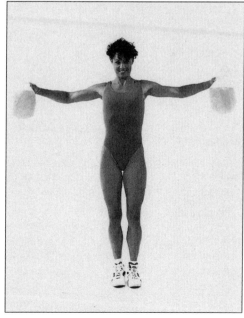

Upright Row (end)

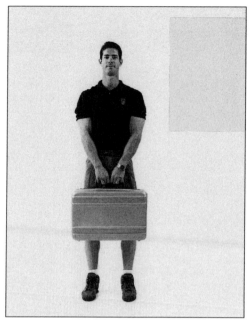

Side Lateral Raise (begin)

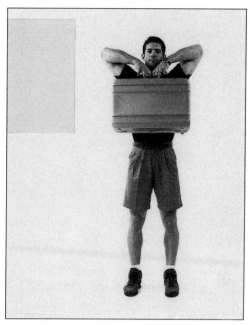

Side Lateral Raise (end)

PROPER POSTURE WHILE MOVING, STANDING OR SITTING

First, let's talk about posture and support of the body when standing and/or sitting. Just so we agree on terms, posture simply means the position or alignment of a body part.

Posture as a term is misleading. It suggests a fixed position, such as standing or sitting. To be more correct, posture is really the use of the body in achieving or maintaining any position or movement. That is to say that one can have good posture even while walking or moving. Posture has everything to do with the way the different segments of the body relate to one another, whether moving or in a static state. Smooth, coordinated control of one's muscles relates to posture just as much as does standing or sitting nicely. Posture involves the entire body musculature.

In any good posture, either moving or remaining still, the body should feel a sense of the absence of conscious effort. One should not have to consciously "feel" the muscle tension needed to retain good posture. Admittedly, this may take a little bit of time for some people to obtain, especially so if poor posture has been their habit. But it can be done, and usually in only a few days.

When one examines superior athletes in any of the sports, one of the comments heard many times is that "they make it look so easy." And, of course, for them, that is true. They do not have to consciously tell their body to move in a certain fashion. The necessary movements are "second nature" for them – that's why it looks so easy. Fortunately, you and I can take advantage of that second nature as well, as we retrain our bodies into a correct and easy-to-maintain posture.

Proper body alignment (posture) normally most favors function. That is to say that a healthy body desires the position that requires the least muscular work to maintain. By so doing, this puts the least amount of strain on muscles, ligaments, tendons and bones.

GOOD POSTURE

Basically, proper posture demands that we keep the body's center of gravity over its base.

Good posture in a standing position requires that the head and chest are held high, the chin, abdomen and buttocks are pulled in, the knees are bent slightly with the feet placed firmly on the ground about shoulder width apart.

Since gravity tends to pull against various parts of the body, the bones, being irregularly shaped, must balance themselves on one another. Gravity pulls the bones downward against each other. So, the only way that the body can be held upright is for the muscles to exert a continual pull on the bones in the opposite direction of gravity.

Gravity pulls the head and trunk forward and downward. The muscles, head and trunk extenders must therefore be pulled backward and upward. For instance, gravity pulls the lower jaw downward; muscles must pull it upward.

The following exercises will help you achieve good posture in the Frontal trunk muscle groups.

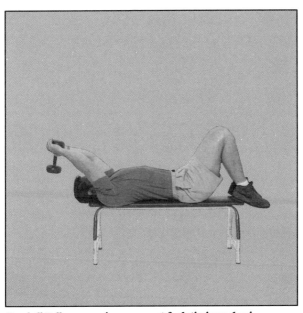

Dumbell Pullover exercise movement for latissimus dorsi

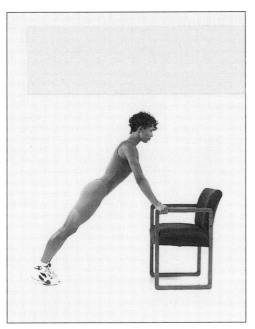

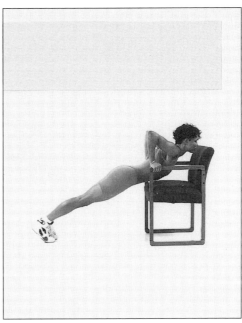

Easy Pushup (begin) *Easy Pushup (end)*

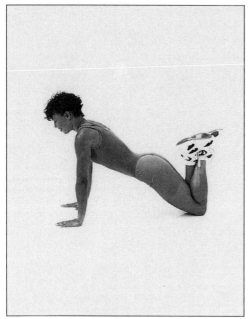

Medium Pushup (begin)

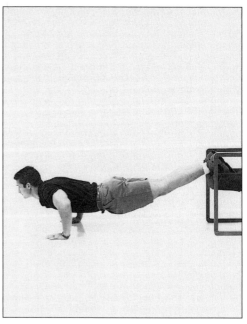

Medium Pushup (end)

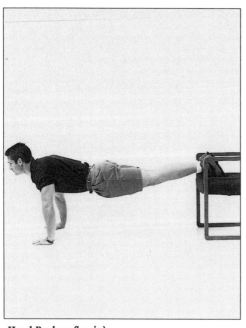

Hard Pushup (begin)

Hard Pushup (end)

Muscles exert this pull using the property of tonicity, or muscle tone. Because tonicity is absent during sleep, muscles cannot counteract the pull of gravity. That's why we can't sleep standing up. Incidentally, the nervous system is also partially responsible for muscle tone, and regulates and coordinates the amount of pull exerted by the individual muscles.

The structures of the muscles and bones play an important part in maintaining good posture. Respiratory, digestive, circulatory and expiratory muscle groups all contribute toward the ability of muscles to maintain posture. This is one of the many examples of the important principle of all body functions being interdependent.

The importance of posture can perhaps be best evaluated by considering some of the effects of poor posture. Poor posture causes the muscles to work harder to counteract the pull of gravity. This quickly leads to fatigue. Good posture requires less muscle strength, and thus less energy demand, than poor posture.

Poor posture also puts more strain on the ligaments. It puts abnormal strains on the bone and may eventually produce structural integration problems and possibly even osteoarthritis. Poor posture also interferes with various bodily functions such as respiration, heart action and digestion.

Practice walking and standing stretched out as high vertically as you can go. Try to imagine a broom handle in your back – walk tall and erect. Do this every time you remember it, and soon you'll be on your way to doing it subconsciously.

When sitting, don't slouch. Slouching in a chair pushes out your stomach. Make sure your feet touch the ground. If you're too short for this to work, either lower the height of your chair or try putting a small pillow behind your back. This brings your torso forward and you shouldn't have to slump down to get your legs over the edge of the chair.

As they say in the military, suck in your gut and stick out your chest. Pulling in the tummy raises the rib cage and gives our internal organs more room. It also stops the rib cage from collapsing onto the abdominals and pushing them out. So, you'll look better and feel better. It's important to do this every time you remember so you train your body to naturally seek out this correct posture on its own.

POOR POSTURE CAUSES OTHER HEALTH PROBLEMS TOO

The mechanical efficiency for any functional design depends upon a centered axis. This is most important for proper posture. However, the human body has a tendency to resist a unified centered axis, largely because it's a flexible, moving structure. In this case, our bodies take the path of least resistance and accept whatever posture is easiest for them to maintain. That posture can be either helped by strong, flexible muscles or hindered by weak, tight muscles.

Poor posture even affects how well we breathe. And as we'll see, how we breathe affects many areas of our lives.

Simply stated, we knew how to breathe correctly at birth. Not coincidentally, babies have the unique ability to both swallow and breathe through the mouth at the same time. Babies are born nose-breathers, inhaling and exhaling through the nose almost all the time, except when crying or nursing.

Abnormal posture is evident in patients with chronic pain-related conditions including backache, headache and stress-related illnesses. Posture training and gravity-centered breathing may play a role in comprehensive treatment of patients with chronic pain and stress-related problems.

There is much evidence to indicate that one's posture can affect body physiology and function. Observations of the striking influence of postural mechanics on function and symptomatology have led to our hypothesis that posture affects and moderates every physiologic function from breathing to hormonal production.

Spinal pain, headache, mood, blood pressure, pulse and lung capacity are among the functions most easily influenced by posture. The most significant influences of posture are upon respiration, oxygenation and sympathetic function. Ultimately, it appears that homeostasis and autonomic regulation are intimately connected with posture. The corollary of these observations is that many symptoms, including pain, may be moderated or eliminated by improved posture.

In terms of body mechanics, posture is more fully defined as the interrelationship between muscle and the skeletal tissue of the body. As Bunch states, "For many years physiologists have shown that the position of the head on the neck is vital because it governs all postural reflexes. If the head is misaligned, other parts of the body move in and out of line to maintain balance and thus energy is expended to counteract the effects of gravity."

Most people, because of poor posture, do not ventilate and oxygenate their bodies optimally. On the other hand, those persons standing straight and tall invariably exude vitality and project a commanding vocal presence. Even that elusive attribute enviably referred to as charisma may well be nothing more than a state of mind reflected in the postural, visual and audio presence of those few individuals with properly-adjusted postures.

Numerous authors have considered some aspects of posture, muscle, tension and/or oxygenation. According to Freeman, shifts in centers of gravity or postural adjustments of aging lead to intestinal diverticula, hemorrhoids, varicosities of the legs, osteoporosis, hip and foot deformities, overall poorer health and even shortened life span. Freeman further theorizes that carbon dioxide retention is partly responsible for many of these changes.

The energetics of skeletal muscle, sensation, circulation, bone growth, fat deposits, immune function, hormonal functions and even enzyme activity are all sympathetically influenced functions. The best known effect of sympathicotonia upon pain is reflex sympathetic dystrophy, but vasospasm and other trophic influences of a "facilitated" (hyper-excitable) neuronal pool affect sensation and muscle tension.

Muscle tension throughout the body is modulated by sympathetic activity which, in turn, is related to all aspects of posture. In summary, the focal stress of spinal misalignment leads to muscle tension, hyperesthesia, altered circulation and a wide variety of visceral illnesses generally associated with stress.

Reich included posture and respiration in his concepts of health. For instance, he believed that tension led to decreased blood flow and that this decrease in tissue oxygenation was a major factor in disease, including cancer. Funderbunk has reported significant evidence of the influence of breathing upon sympathetic function, physiology and catecholamine production, although he does not include posture as a major modulator of breathing.

GOOD POSTURE HELPS PREVENT HEALTH PROBLEMS

At the Shealy Institute, clinicians have consistently observed striking postural abnormalities in virtually every patient with back pain, headache or depression. The Institute clinicians' observations of postural abnormalities noted in 27 consecutive headache patients follow. There were 21 women age 18-69 and six men age 31-57. Eleven of the 26 patients had migraines. Sixteen had significant myofascial pain, often post-whiplash or post-cervical fusion.

Twenty six patients had various postural abnormalities, with only one migrainous patient exhibiting normal posture. The postural abnormalities noted included a wide variety of abnormalities – a total of 131 postural deviations in 26 patients. The most common were:

Compressed or flattened thoracic spine	20
Head forward	17
Increased lordosis	11
Kyphosis	9
Scoliosis	9
Rotated pelvis	9

Additionally, several patients exhibited rotation of head, shoulders, legs and feet. Thus, postural abnormalities seem to contribute some degree of autonomic, myotonic and sensory facilitation in most patients with headache; even modest improvements in posture often assist patients in achieving greater comfort. Optimizing posture and respiration should lead to even more striking improvement.

This and other personal observations have led us to the conclusion that optimal posture and its accompanying improved respiratory/oxygenation offer potentially powerful influences upon autonomic nervous system function.

Numerous individuals have reported improvement in a variety of illnesses after practice of proper breathing. Back pain, headache, TMJ syndrome, depression, hypertension, asthma, anxiety – all stress illnesses – have responded favorably in non-controlled application of proper breathing.

CONCLUSION

1. Posture affects all human function, both consciously and unconsciously, from breathing to thinking.

2. Because posture affects breathing, it also influences vocal sound. If sound is not optimally vocalized, the individual does not experience optimal vocal expression.

3. Posture reflects mind and body interaction. Inefficient postural and resultant poor breathing habits eventually lead, in extreme cases, to pathologic dysfunction.

4. Individuals in advanced stages of postural/breathing dysfunction often suffer from structural deviations so marked as to impede efficient air exchange and elicit a sympathetic nervous system stress response, as well as increased musculoskeletal pain.

5. Maximally efficient breathing and posture open pathways to body-mind balance and improved well-being. The more effectively one breathes, the greater overall health.

6. Postural/respiratory balance and improved homeostasis can be taught through proper physiologic breathing techniques.[202]

How To Correct Your Abdomen Bulge Caused By Pelvic Shift After Pregnancy

I t is almost a universally accepted axiom that women gain weight and keep it on after pregnancy. There's just one problem with the axiom — it's not true. At least, it doesn't need to be.

There are simply too many ways for a woman to get fit and stay fit, and too many benefits to remaining strong and well-exercised throughout a pregnancy.

First, it is very important that a woman develop good muscle tone and cardiorespiratory fitness before she becomes pregnant. That alone should solve most of the problems and discomforts associated with being pregnant. A well-toned body is able to cope with increased physical and emotional demands much better than an out-of-shape couch potato.

And it needs to be said that a woman who isn't pregnant can pretty much do any exercise routine that she wants to. Her only limitation is her mental attitude and muscle exhaustion level.

That is not true of a woman after she's pregnant. While the limits imposed on her are not severe, there are still some things that she probably cannot do, for her safety and that of the baby.

Having said that, *Muscle & Fitness* magazine followed Beth Deters and her workout schedule throughout her pregnancy. Beth emphatically stated, "There's just no reason a woman has to lose her body because of motherhood. I see so many women today who maintain a regular exercise regimen right up until delivery. They look and feel terrific all the way through their pregnancies, and within weeks [after delivery] their bodies are back to being fit and fabulous." [204]

As the magazine chronicled, Mrs. Deters remained on her regular exercise routine throughout her pregnancy with just a few minor alterations.

While Beth was able to continue doing leg exercises, many women find that uncomfortable. The hip and pelvic joints are becoming more pliable and flexible. That makes leg and hip exercises, such as squats and lunges, uncomfortable for many women. So much so that some women find they need to be more careful in guarding against falls even while walking or using the stairs.

The end result of Beth's pregnancy workouts: a very respectable 20 pound weight gain and a healthy baby girl, Brenna Sloan Deters.

Even while pregnant, it's important to maintain some sort of modest physical exercise. Walking is good as it works both aerobically to keep the weight down and also as a general muscle toner. You can also get some upper body workout if you walk with small handheld weights.

With the doctor's permission, you might also want to try low-impact aerobics. It works well, and doesn't overdo those now-flexible and unstable lower body joints.

These same exercises, continued as soon after pregnancy as your doctor approves, also help to even out hormonal surges and reduce or eliminate the postpartum letdown "blues."

Regaining your flat tummy, cinched-in waist and torso subtleness following pregnancy is dependent upon proper exercises and understanding the body changes brought on by and during the pregnancy.

For, after months of increasing pressure on the stomach by the baby, abdominal muscles are stretched to the limit. Their functions are varied to accommodate the growing baby.

Elizabeth Noble, author of Essential Exercises for the Childbearing Years, is the founder of the Obstetrics and Gynecology Section of the American Physical Therapy Association. She included obstetrics and gynecology as part of the curriculum during her studies of physiotherapy in her native Adeliade, Australia.

Noble takes great care in describing the various functions of the abdominal muscles which she compares to an elaborate corset.

"Although each segment of the abdominal corset makes a key contribution, during exercises and activities the different parts are combined rather than isolated," she writes. "For example, the top half of the corset is emphasized during movements with the upper trunk; the lower abdominals work to stabilize the pelvis when the legs are moved."

These muscles are not exercised enough, she says, because of the habit of standing, sitting or "walking at a normal pace on level ground. The abdominals are usually the weakest group of muscles among the general population and their weakness is one of the most common causes of backache," And that's without a pregnancy.[205]

The pregnancy places extra demands on the abdominal muscles which must then bear the increasing size of the uterus. "Evidence of this is also seen superficially by stretch marks which indicate that the skin has reached the limit of its elasticity," Noble points out. It also obliterates the navel, "which occurs around the seventh month."

The muscles must be kept in good shape during the pregnancy so that they can support the baby, which, at the same time, is adding pressure to the backbone.

The following exercises will help you both before and after pregnancy.

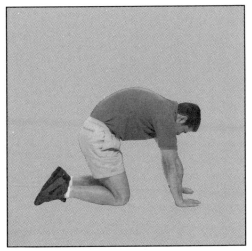

Kneeling Back Arch for stretching erector spinae (low back)

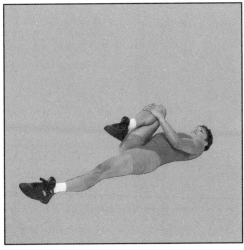

Single Knee to Chest Stretch for low back muscles (erector spinae, gluteus maximus)

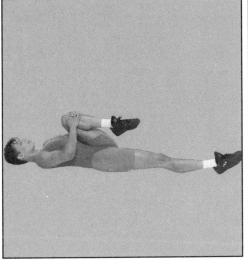

Single Knee to Chest Stretch, different camera angle

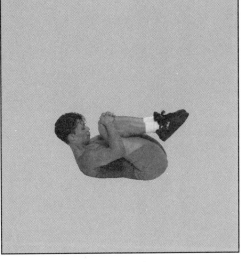

Double Knee to Chest Stretch

31

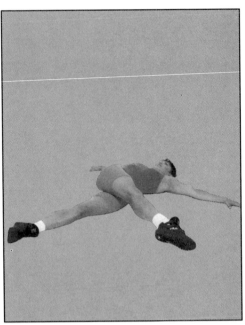

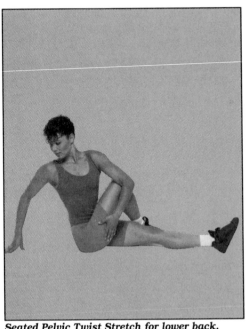

Lying Pelvic Twist Stretch for lower back, obliques and gluteus maximus

Seated Pelvic Twist Stretch for lower back, obliques and gluteus maximus

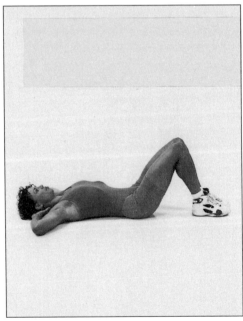

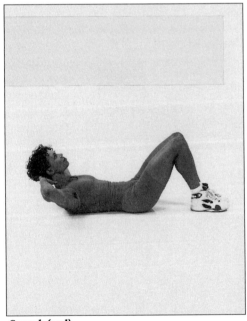

Crunch (begin)

Crunch (end)

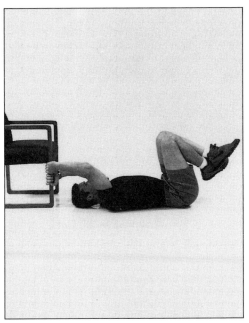

Tuck (begin)

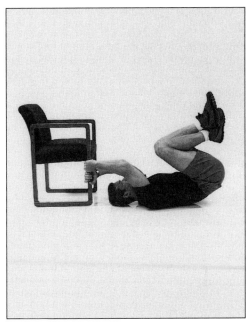

Tuck (end)

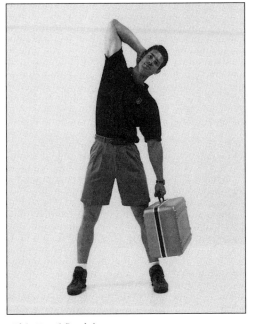

Side Bend (begin)

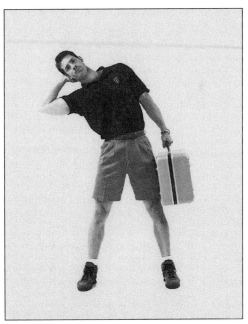

Side Bend (end)
(Switch and do other side also.)

The solution to this, according to Noble is "a correct pelvic tilt. Without it, poor posture, muscle strain and backache result. The abdominal muscles feel deceivingly fit during pregnancy because they are being continuously stretched over the enlarging uterus — the resistance keeps them taut. Because they are stretched so tight, it is important to avoid any positions or exercises that cause further stretch or the muscles will be weakened," Noble states.

Following delivery, or postpartum, there needs to be a time for the muscles to return to their normal positions. Some of this is automatic, but exercises are called for to return other muscles to normalcy.

"Muscles do recover their inherent properties, and exercise during pregnancy will facilitate recovery afterward," Noble advises, adding, "Supple muscles, which have maintained their contractile ability and blood circulation as much as possible, will lengthen more easily and shorten more quickly afterward."

It is recommended that special exercises be taken during pregnancy. Also, these now are being offered by the YMCA's and private exercise studios following pregnancy.

However, it is not recommended to use the same sets of exercises for both periods of time. During postpartum strains on the backbone or abdominal muscles stretching has to be avoided.

"The ligaments will gradually tighten back to their former stage as the uterus returns to normal due to the physiological adjustments of the body during the post-partum weeks," Nobel says.

But, "returning the abdominal muscles to their former shape, size and efficiency requires the mother's active input with best results achieved when exercises are commenced within 24 hours after delivery," Noble said.

Other tips from the author are:

- "Exercise in pregnancy or even before should be commenced as early as possible so that the new mother has achieved the minimum normal strength levels before the muscles start to stretch."

- Since the abdominal muscles have been subjected to prolonged tension stress, it is important not to overwork them;

- Strong exercises must not be attempted until there has been a good recovery of the abdominal wall and pelvic floor which varies "with each woman and relates to her physical condition before pregnancy, her labor and delivery as well as the management in the immediate postpartum phase."

Sylvia Klein Olkin, author of both <u>Positive Pregnancy Fitness</u> and <u>Positive Parenting Fitness</u>, explains the changes in the mother's body during pregnancy:

"The center of gravity gradually changes. Before pregnancy, the body weight is centered over the hips, but as the baby grows, the center of gravity shifts so most of the mother's weight is in front of her hips. This leads to changes in the arrangement of her spine. The natural S-curve deepens and the vertebrae change position as the weight on the front of the belly increases. After childbirth, the goal is to gradually return the spine to its prepregnancy alignment."

There also is the goal to regain the muscle tone of prepregnancy. This may take a while, the author points out.

Olkin shares these tips:

- During pregnancy and right after delivery, joints are more flexible and less secure. It may take three to six months or more for these bodily changes to revert back to normal.

- If good posture was maintained during the pregnancy, the mother may have fewer complaints after giving birth.

- If the mother exercised and did light weight training during her pregnancy, she should have a much easier time getting back into shape because she has maintained appropriate muscle tone.

- The body has amazing powers of rejuvenation and the overstretched, overworked muscles will shorten and become more elastic if the mother makes a conscious effort to feel the muscles she is using when holding a proper posture.

- It takes from three to six months for most women's bodies to adjust to the non-pregnant state and up to nine months to fully recover from pregnancy and childbirth.

- For approximately six months after the birth of the baby, the mother's joints will be more flexible and less secure. It may take up to six months or more for her body to revert back to normal.

- According to a number of exercise physiologists, a proper, safe and effective workout combines three separate components that are practiced in a proper sequence: warm-up stage, low-impact aerobics and a cool-down period.[206]

For more specific information on fitness and pregnancy, you might want to contact Sylvia Klein Olkin, founder of Positive Pregnancy and Parenting Fitness, 51 Saltrock Road, Baltic, CT 06330. Her toll-free telephone number is 800-433-5523.

5

How To Correct Your Abdomen Bulge Caused By Poor Breathing

I t appears to be inconceivable that one can get a flat tummy, a cinched-in waist and firm buttocks just by breathing.

If that is the case, why don't we all have just that? After all, we all breathe and, according to Webster, to breathe is the ability to take air into the lungs and expel it from the lungs — to inhale and to exhale. It is an automatic function that generally we don't even think about doing.

So, how could the simple act of breathing firm up the waist and buttocks, and flatten the tummy? What have we not been told?

The simple fact is that there are a number of different ways to breathe and there are experts who point out these various "ways" in order to get the most out of a lungful of air. However, with all of the excellent information and theories they provide, they don't seem to conscientiously make the effort to combine breathing with muscle tightening.

One of the experts is Ian Jackson, author of The Breathplay Approach to Wholelife Fitness, who writes of his perfected proper way to breathe. Another is Carola H. Speads, a renowned expert on breathing work and author of Breathing: The ABC's, who maintains that there are many different ways to breathe.[207]

Both of them, in presenting their theories, offer exercises which involve many of the muscles that have gone flabby.

In studying these two authors' accounts of how to breathe properly, there is one curious similarity. The fact remains that a side effect of breathing properly results in a certain amount of muscle tightening and strengthening right where it's needed.

Jackson is a fitness expert who has served as a trainer for both Olympic athletes and corporate executives and as a triathlon competitor. He has been in a position to see the effects of different ways of breathing, having served as a special coach/advisor to 7-Eleven's America's Team, the first American bicycling team to enter the Tour de France in 1986. But he doesn't confine his instructions to the intensive athlete or fitness person. He reaches out to all people interested in improving their health.

While most people believe that inbreath (inhaling) is where they should place their greatest breathing effort and treat outbreath (exhaling) as an automatic process, Jackson says that he has found just the opposite — that outbreathing is where the emphasis should be and that inhaling should follow without effort.

He says that by using this method, one has more strength in his command. Jackson suggests a concerted effort be made to tuck the buttocks tightly in, squeeze the abdominal muscles and "swoosh" the exhale breath out of the lungs. Then, he says, relax and let the new air enter the lungs normally without sucking it in, which he terms this inhaling process as passive entry.

He advocates that an easy way of learning this method is to think of breathing as a stomach-flattening technique. Push the air out by flattening the belly. Relax and passively let the air enter. That is the basis of his teaching. He also points out that if one does it consistently enough, inches will disappear from the waist.

Logic backs this premise. The tightening of pelvic and stomach muscles causes the rubber-band-like muscle action to tighten.

People without an excess of fat still can have flabby muscle mass. As they begin to breathe in a controlled manner, they are strengthening the muscles. The tighter the muscles the tighter they cling to the body

Therefore it is logical that the relationship between the muscles used in breathing and the surrounding muscles that also have other functions, when properly conditioned, have a direct bearing on controlling the tummy and lower abdomen.

The exercises on the following pages will help strengthen the various muscle groups needed for good breathing.

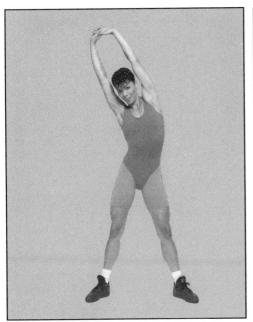

Standing Side Bend Stretch for upper back and rib cage, latissimus dorsi, intercostals and serratus anterior

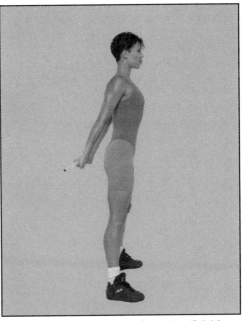

Rear Shoulder Stretch for anterior and medial deltoids and pectoral major

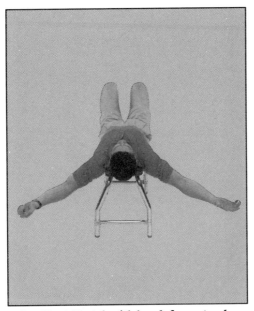

Lying Chest Stretch with bench for pectoral major, serratus anterior and intercostals

39

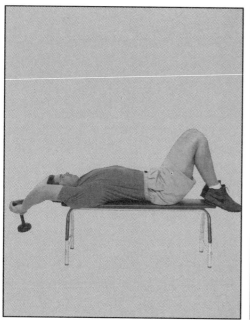

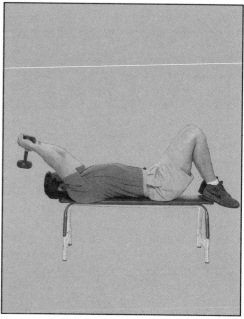

Dumbell Pullover exercise movement for latis-simus dorsi, pectoralis major, intercostals and serratus anterior (begin)

Dumbell Pullover (middle)

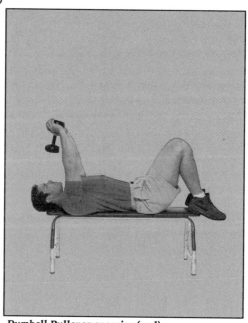

Dumbell Pullover exercise (end)

According to Jackson, the lungs "have no muscle at all. Were it not for the help of other muscles, they would be unable to pump air and thus unable to deliver oxygen to the body and to remove carbon dioxide from it.

"For the lungs to pump air, the muscles of the rib cage and diaphragm must work together to alternately squeeze and open the surrounding space," the author points out.

Jackson's description of the duties of the diaphragm, the rib cage and belly illustrates the importance of keeping these body parts in top operational form while they attend to the important duty of governing the breathing process, while offering an obvious solution of tightening those pesky "loose" and undisciplined muscles to keep us taut and springboard fit.

"The diaphragm works within the body the way a piston works within a cylinder," Jackson explains. "To squeeze the lungs and thus push air out, the diaphragm domes up into the rib cage like a piston pushing up into a cylinder. To create the partial vacuum that will draw the lungs open again, it then flattens down into the abdominal cavity.

"This up-and-down movement is not exactly like that of a piston within a cylinder because our bodies are so much more wonderfully made than are engines," he continues. "Both the cylinder and the piston of our air pump change shape as they work together. The rib cage closes in on itself as the diaphragm domes up into it, and it opens up as the diaphragm flattens down."

"We have conscious control of the rib cage and belly muscles, but not of the diaphragm," he says.

Jackson points out that there are people who have extra weight in their midsection or weak muscles in the abdominal wall. By changing their breathing technique, they are finding that the midsection tightens up and the muscles in the abdominal wall are pulling their tummies flat. One of the rewards of proper breathing, he explains.

Also, abdominal exercises like the ones pictured will build abdominal and diaphragm strength.

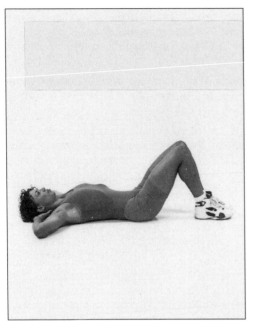

Crunch (begin)

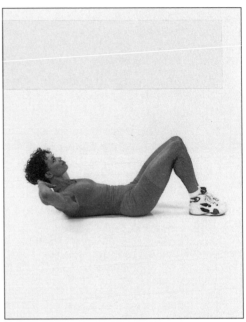

Crunch (end)

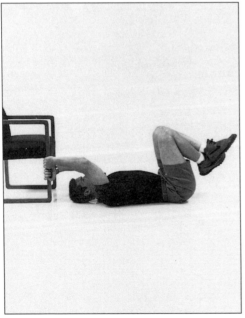

Tuck (begin)

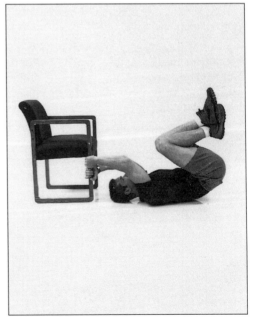

Tuck (end)

Speads, while addressing breathing differently than Jackson, says that "breathing, unlike other involuntary functions, is also partially under the influence of the voluntary nervous system. Muscles, tendons and joints have an influence on it."

Speads, who has taught breathing classes both in the United States and abroad, believes that there is no one way of breathing that is the right way or the best way to be aimed for at all times.

"We breathe in many ways," she says, "and many ways of breathing may be appropriate. Breathing is right not when it functions all the time in one particular 'ideal' manner, but when it works in a way that lets it freely adjust, changing its quality according to our needs of the moment."

Many of her breathing exercises, while ostensibly are for better breathing habits, also stretch the body's muscles, toning them to support the process of "various breathing techniques" and at the same time streamline the muscular structure of the body.

"Running requires a different kind of breathing from sleeping," she points out, while "alertness for an important interview is of a different quality of breathing from that for a casual chat with a friend. Anger will make us breathe differently from serenity. A certain kind of breathing may be right for one situation, but inadequate for another." And, "Sometimes a very full breath will be appropriate; other times a much shallower one."

Even the casual reader of breathing techniques absorbs the underlying thread that breathing exercises are also muscle strengthening exercises.

6

The Campitelli Advanced Abdomen Reduction and Stretching Method

Using new scientific principles of resistance training, it is no longer necessary to endure hours of brutal gut-wrenching workouts in order to have a fit and toned body. In fact, it can be done quickly and easily in only minutes a week.

Throughout Part One, you've seen various stretches and exercises to help build muscle strength. Some photos may have been in more than one section since my method uses dynamic whole-body movements that exercise several muscle groups at the same time.

For your ease of use during actual workouts, the stretches and exercises are pictured here in their entirety.

Now, let's demonstrate the stomach and muscle toning exercises.

ABDOMEN REDUCTION EXERCISES

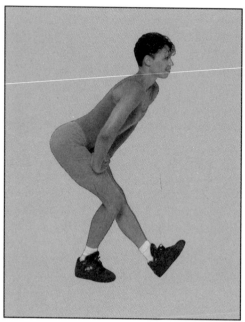

Fig. 1- Standing Stretch for hamstring group (left leg stretch)

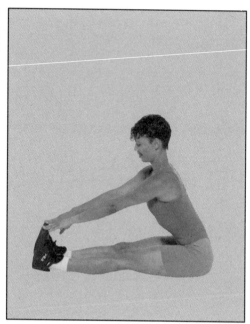

Fig. 2 - Seated Double Hamstring Stretch (both legs)

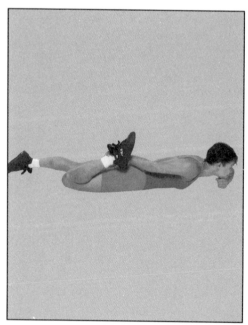

Fig. 3 - Lying Quadricep Stretch for elongating quadricep (thigh) muscle

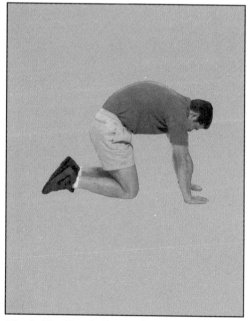

Fig. 4 - Kneeling Back Arch for stretching erector spinae (low back)

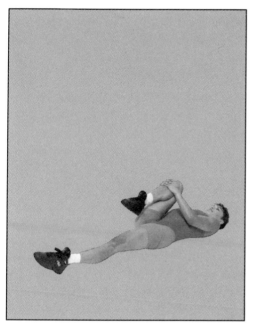

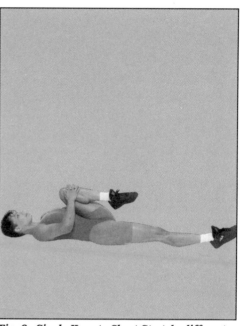

Fig. 5 - *Single Knee to Chest Stretch for low back muscles (erector spinae, gluteus maximus)*

Fig. 6 - *Single Knee to Chest Stretch, different camera angle*

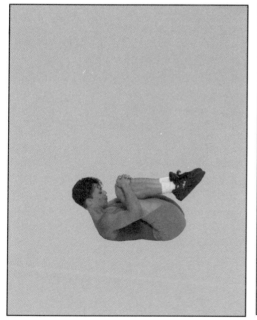

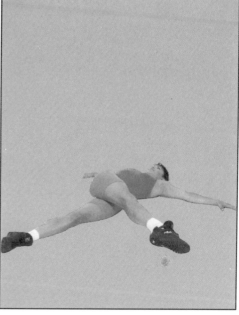

Fig. 7 - *Double Knee to Chest Stretch (exercises same muscle groups as #5)*

Fig. 8 - *Lying Pelvic Twist Stretch for lower back, obliques and gluteus maximus*

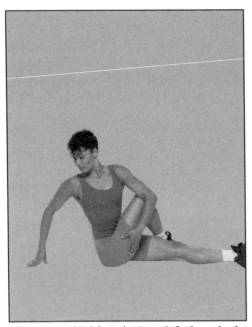

Fig. 9 - Seated Pelvic Twist Stretch for lower back, obliques and gluteus maximus

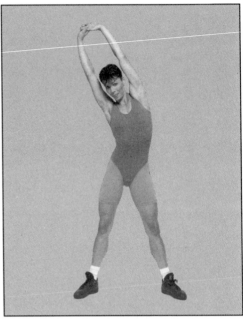

Fig. 10 - Standing Side Bend Stretch for upper back and rib cage, latissimus dorsi, inter-costals and serratus anterior

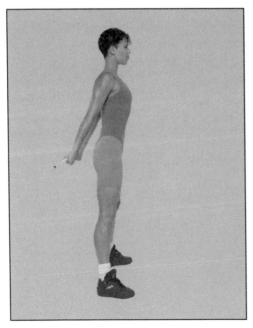

Fig. 11 - Rear Shoulder Stretch for anterior and medial deltoids and pectoral major

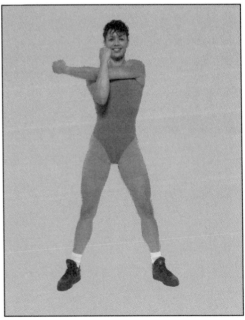

Fig. 12 - Front Shoulder Stretch for upper back trapezius, rhomboids and posterior deltoid

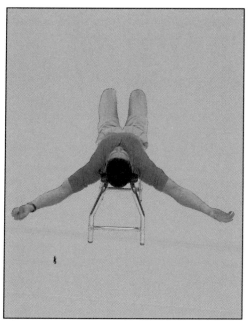

Fig. 13 - Lying Chest Stretch with bench for pectoral major, serratus anterior and intercostals

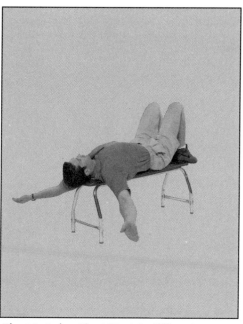

Fig. 14 - Lying Chest Stretch, different camera angle

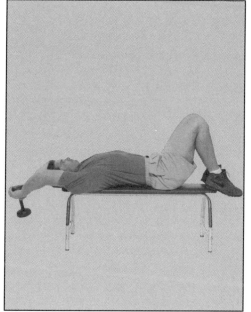

Fig. 15A - Dumbell Pullover exercise movement for latissimus dorsi, pectoralis major, intercostals and serratus anterior (begin)

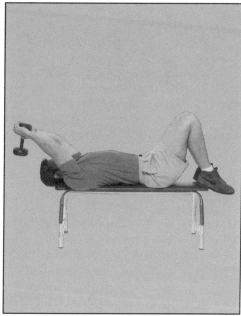

Fig. 15B - Dumbell Pullover (middle)

49

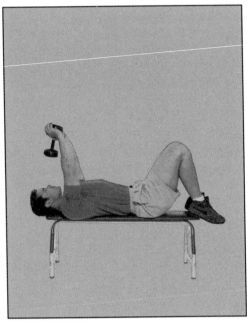

Fig. 15C - Dumbell Pullover exercise (end)

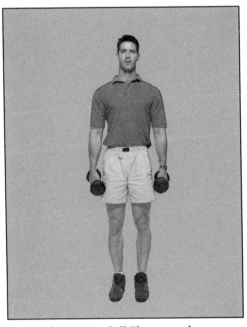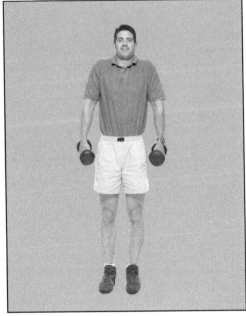

Fig. 16 - Dumbell Shrug exercise movement for trapezius muscle

Getting rid of that tummy really depends on two factors — controlling the appetite and exercising the proper muscles. Contrary to what most of us think, appetite control is really quite easy. So, before we outline the revolutionary Campitelli Method, let's discuss a few hints and tips for eating less to help get rid of excess interabdominal fat.

A simple beginning hint is this: drink more water to fill up your tummy. Drink a large glass of water shortly before each meal, and drink between meals too.

Many times, what we perceive as hunger is not hunger at all, but rather thirst. Much of the food we eat doesn't contain very much water. And often, we don't drink enough water throughout the day.

Yes, the standard prescription for those obligatory 8 glasses of water a day is quite true. If we fill up on water, which has zero calories and no fat, we'll likely eat less food and yet be fully satisfied.

Eat small amounts of food throughout the day. Eat, eat, and eat some more. But go easy on it – a small handful of food is really just enough. This keeps the metabolism stoked and really burns up the calories. Concentrate on vegetables, a few fruits and plenty of complex carbohydrates (whole grains, rice, pasta and the like).

Skip the appetizers, or have a cup of a broth-based soup. Stay away from cream-based soups since they're usually high in fat.

Eat more spicy foods. The jolt from the flavor satisfies our appetites more quickly. And if you can eat food spicy enough to make you sweat, you've just boosted your metabolic rate skyward, and supercharged your tummy-losing potential!

Be sure to follow the Biotech Low-Fat eating suggestions. Our bodies can store 100,000 or more calories of fat, but only about 2,000 calories of carbohydrates. Digesting carbohydrates increases the metabolic rate, while digesting fat decreases the metabolic rate. And those fat calories speed along to almost immediate storage on our belly, hips and thighs.

Here's another appetite decreasing tip: eat whole grain bread about 20 minutes or so before the main course. This gives the complex carbos time to reach your hypothalamus and turn off your appetite. Imagine — by the time you're done with bread (no butter please!) and salad, you'll feel absolutely stuffed. And you'll eat much less. And you'll lose that belly.

THE CAMPITELLI ADVANCED METHOD - EXERCISING AND STRETCHING

As we've already discussed, there are various causes for a bulging abdomen. Many of those causes are related to posture and certain muscle groups, not to excess abdominal fat. The Campitelli Advanced Method is solely designed to build up those muscle groups, thereby improving posture and pulling the stomach in. The following information details the importance of each of those muscle groups.

ABDOMINALS

Simply stated, the function of the abdominals is merely to bend the torso either forward or down. If you are lying down, the abdominals pull the rib cage to the groin area, flexing the torso forward.

The thinner lower abdomen muscles must be built up to match the stronger upper abdomen muscles. These also include the external and internal oblique muscles, which are the side or lower torso side muscles.

Exercises that work these muscles are twisting exercises, such as body twists, side crunches and side bends. Some exercise machines also do rotational resistance against these muscle groups. Other exercises that build the abdominals are crunches, tucks and pelvic tilts.

HAMSTRINGS

Another muscle group that needs to be strengthened is the hamstring group.

The hamstrings are connected to the back of the leg and the back of the pelvis. They are used to pull the pelvis back down into a normal position.

Strengthening the hamstrings plays a large part in rotating the pelvis back into the normal position.

MUSCLE TONE

The following is a striking illustration: when a person loses consciousness, muscles lose their tone, and a person collapses into a heap. Unconscious people are unable to maintain any kind of a sitting or standing posture. This is due to tonic contraction or tone, which is a continued partial contraction of the muscle.

At any one moment, a small number of the total muscle fibers contract, producing a tautness of the muscle rather than a recognizable contraction and movement. Different groups of fibers scattered throughout the muscle counteract the relays. Tonic contraction or muscle tone is a basic characteristic of anatomy in individuals when they are awake.

When weight training or some other type of resistance training is introduced, it subjects the muscle fibers to new stresses. As a result, the muscles become larger and more toned. The added benefit of toned muscles is an improvement in posture.

For instance, if a person doesn't have good muscle tone in their upper back, it is hard for them to maintain good posture. The back muscles are not able to counteract the effects of gravity for an extended period of time, and the body begins to slump forward.

BACK

The main muscles involved in strengthening the upper back are the trapezius, rear deltoid, and medial height of the deltoid, teres minor, teres major, lattisimus dorsi, and rhomboid.

There is also a smaller muscle group involved called the levator scapulae.

The exercises which work these separate muscle groups are shoulder shrugs, which strengthen the trapezius (this is the large muscle in the upper back and neck) by simply letting the shoulders drop and pulling the shoulder girdle to the ear.

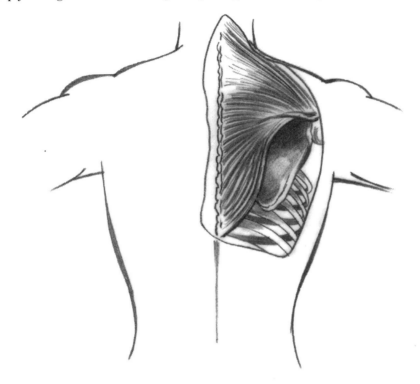

Fig. 6-17

Lateral raises with dumbbells to the side, which moves the upper arm up and away from the side and towards the head. This exercises several different muscles including the trapezius, rhomboids, rear deltoid, and medial head of the deltoid (the shoulder muscle).

Rear deltoid raises, done lying on your stomach while raising your arms up and back, build the mid-to-lower part of the trapezius, rhomboids and rear deltoids.

Pulldowns, rows and chin-ups help the large muscles in the upper back, namely the lats, rhomboids, teres major, teres minor, rear deltoid and trapezius.

Upright rows, done in a standing position and pulling an object from the thigh to the ear position, works the deltoids, trapezius, rhomboids and biceps.

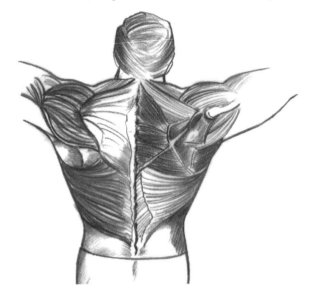

Fig 6-18

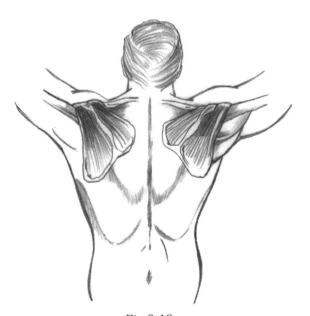

Fig 6-19

Overhead presses work the trapezius and deltoids. These muscles in the upper back will pull the shoulders back and the head up and the chin in, thus reducing the sag in the slump of the shoulders, which collapses the lungs and diaphragm area. As we've already seen, collapsing the rib cage down against the abdomen is a major cause of a protruding belly.

The lower back curve, called the lordotic curve, must not be allowed to get into a "swayback" position. The chest must not cave in with the shoulders drooping forward. The head and neck cannot drop onto the chest, or shorten up and settle back into the shoulders.

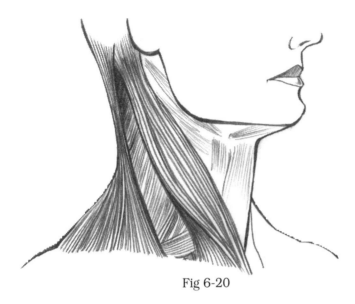

Fig 6-20

The back is most protected, and most efficient, when the normal back curves are maintained like we had when we were young. It can then protect you and allow you the fullest range of motion, whether you are walking, sitting, bending, playing sports, exercising or doing any of your favorite activities.

Muscle tissue makes up nearly half of your body weight. Important to a healthy back are the abdominal muscles. They reach all the way from the sternum in the front down to the pubic bone. Healthy abdominal muscles greatly reduce the likelihood of back pain and problems. Along with the abdominals, other muscles in the upper back, shoulder, sides, neck and thighs activate and/or protect the back muscles by reducing the muscle force needed for the back muscles to accomplish work or by limiting the range of motion.[203]

STRETCHING

Besides exercise, the other half of the equation important for reducing the size of our abdomens is stretching. Above all, it increases the range of motion of the frontal areas of the body.

Simply stated, weak muscles need to be strengthened, and strong muscles need to be stretched. Stretching is an important component of any fitness regimen. Unfortunately, it's often the most over looked aspect of fitness. We have the mistaken notion that if we exercise a muscle for strength, it's gotten all the stretching it needs.

Not so. Strong muscles need to be flexible as well as powerful, and stretching is the only way to accomplish that goal.

There are two types of stretching techniques. Active stretching uses the muscle force of the individual to stretch the muscle. In passive stretching, a partner supplies the force on the muscle.

Static stretching is the most popular form of active stretches. The individual simply moves into a comfortable stretch and holds that position for the desired time. This is the safest technique, and the one I recommend for beginners.

Ballistic stretching is still an active stretch, but substitutes bouncing and rapid movements for the static hold. The risk of muscle injury is greater in ballistic stretching than the static mode, so be very careful. Beginners should not do ballistic stretches. Get a bit developed in both muscle strength and static stretching first before you venture into the ballistic method.

First, a few important directions on stretching. Many people stretch with the intention of becoming more flexible, therefore they stretch the muscle as far as possible. In doing so they constantly over-stretch the muscle. This intense stretch tightens muscles, and causes microscopic tears. This in turn causes scars to form in the muscle fibers. As scars are non-elastic, muscle elasticity is actually reduced, thereby contributing to muscle pain.

This non-elastic dense scar tissue in the muscle fibers interferes with normal blood flow and distribution of nerve input, leaving the muscle and surrounding connective tissues vulnerable to further injury and loss of motion. This vicious cycle is repeated each time over-stretching occurs.

Stretching is important; stretching correctly even more so. The stretch reflex occurs when you put a joint in a dangerous position, such as in a flex or stretch of a muscle group beyond its limit. At this point, the muscle contracts to relieve the stress on the joint so it is no longer in a dangerous position.

When one stretches correctly, the stretch reflexes are not activated in muscles and the tissues are not harmed. Proper stretching elongates the muscle slowly to a point where mild tension is felt.

For an easy stretch, a long position is held for 10-30 seconds, during which time there should be no discomfort. The longer the easy stretch is held, the more elongated the muscle becomes and the less the stretch is " felt." Forcing a stretch beyond the point of mild muscle tension is over-stretching, and one should ease off into a more comfortable position.

The easy stretch is important because it reduces muscle tension, maintains flexibility and reduces or prevents soreness. This easy stretch does not activate the stretch reflex mechanism and should always precede more vigorous stretching in order to increase flexibility.

Stretching to the point of pain activates the tendons and muscle spindle structures, technically called sarcomeres, actin, myosin and Z-discs. Their function in an overstretch is to protect the muscle from damage. So, if you feel pain, you've overstretched, and the muscle will actually lose flexibility in order to protect itself from damage.

Correct stretching avoids pain. The muscle can feel tight, but no pain must be present. Hold this tight position for 10-15 seconds and then release. Stretch again and hold for 20-30 seconds. Concentrate on feeling the muscle relax and lengthen.

Now comes the real benefit. Stretch again and hold 30-60 seconds for the easy stretch. Breathe slowly and deeply through your nose. This third stretch, done when the muscle is warmed up, accomplishes a great deal in added flexibility.

Before you begin stretching, it is vital that the muscles be thoroughly warmed up. Muscles are rather like rubber bands in this regard. If stretched too far when they are cold, they may break. Once warmed up however, they stretch further with more efficiency.

You can warmup by light jogging, massaging the target muscle groups, light calisthenics, aerobics or any other light activity you enjoy that moves your body weight through a space. After warming up for 10 minutes or so, you're ready for a stretching session.

Muscle groups that need to be stretched for improved posture are the pectoral major, pectoral minor, subscapularis, anterior and medial deltoid, anterior and intercostals of the rib cage and diaphragm of the rib cage. Important lower body muscle groups are the quadriceps and hip flexors of the leg.

As these muscles are stretched and become more flexible, an increased range of motion occurs. The muscles that have been strengthened in the upper back can then pull the shoulder gently back and the rib cage out. When the quadriceps are stretched and the hip flexors are stretched, the pelvis can return to a normal position. This is very important for women after pregnancy.

There are also some exercises that can be used to increase the chest volume and stretch the diaphragm. Most useful are pullovers on a bench or floor, or a straight arm pulldown.

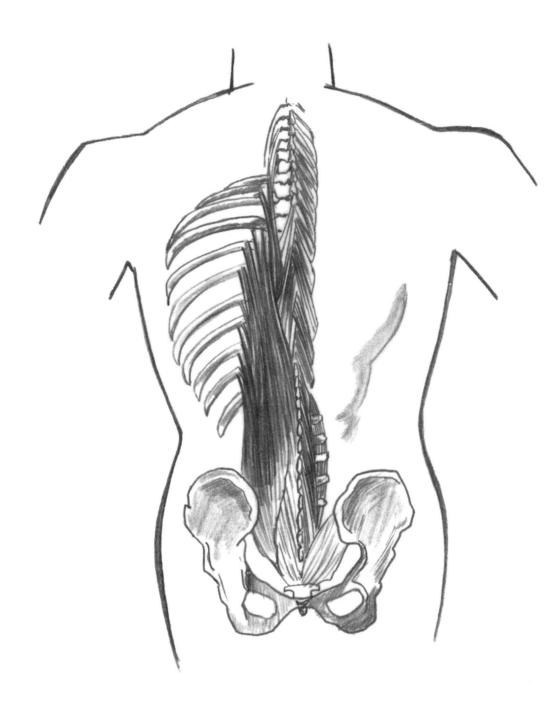

Fig. 6-21

The muscles in the lower back, called the erector spinae, have to be stretched also. As an added benefit for those of you who may be experiencing back pain, exercises and stretches are also indicated to help relieve back pain discomfort.

Chronic back pain also has many of the same causes of a large abdomen, namely poor posture and weak muscles. The techniques we've discussed for stretching the front of your body and the strengthening of your upper back are also related to chronic back pain. Back problems can usually be solved by doing these same exercises and stretches.

All of these exercises can be done in many different styles and resistances, depending on the body position, using machines, weights and other types of exercise devices. All of these exercises are designed to strengthen muscle areas for more support. The more support you have, the more tone you will have. And as we've seen, the more muscle tone, the better your posture and the less problems you will have with untoned muscle groups.

Stretches also increase the amount of fluid in joint cartilages, increase the blood flow to muscles and overall help to warm up the muscles and joints so that the chance of injury is lessened. Warmed and stretched muscles are also able to do more work than tight, cold muscles.

Especially so in the back, weak, tight muscles are very prone to injury. Stretching also helps to increase the range of motion of a joint, very important if you suffer from any kind of arthritis problem.

Above all, stretching should feel good and be fun. Pain, stress or a hard stretching workout imply that you are doing something wrong.

BENEFITS OF STRETCHING

Develops body awareness

Enhances physical fitness

Reduces muscle soreness

Increases skill in various sports

Provides physical and mental relaxation

Reduces the risk of muscle injury

Improves the posture

If you have back problems, or suspect that you might, it is always proper to consult with your health care practitioner before beginning a workout or stretching routine. Additionally, the following resources may prove helpful to you:

The American Academy of Physical Medicine and Rehabilitation
30 North Michigan Ave.
Chicago, IL 60602
312-236-9512

The American Osteopathic Association
212 E. Ohio St.
Chicago, IL 60611
312-280-5800

The American Physical Therapy Association
1111 N. Fairfax St.
Alexandria, VA 22314
703-684-2782

MUSCLE STRETCH ASSESSMENT

The following guidelines will help you determine your present level of muscle flexibility. You can then concentrate stretching routines on the muscle groups that are the least flexible.

Chest and Shoulders

Procedure: Lie flat on the floor on your stomach. Extend arms straight out from your shoulders. Keeping your palms down and arms straight, lift your arms off the floor. Note how far you can lift your arms off the floor and use the following scale:

Poor flexibility - 0-2" elevation

Average flexibility - 2-8" elevation

Good flexibility - more than 8" elevation

Lower Back and Hamstrings

Procedure: Sit on floor with legs extended in front. Keeping legs together and straight, reach for your toes with your hands. Note how far your hands are from your toes and use the following scale:

Poor flexibility - hands more than 10" from toes

Below average flexibility - hands 5-10" from toes

Average flexibility - hands 0-5" from toes

Excellent flexibility - hands reach past your toes

Part Two

How To Get Rid of Excess Fat in the Abdomen and Waist By Actually Eating 400% More and Better Tasting Food

— Plus —

How To Increase Your Body's Fat Burning Rate By 200% to 300%, Sculpture Your Entire Body and Become Much Healthier

7

EAT MORE FOOD AND LOSE WEIGHT

Anyone who has ever been on a restricted calorie diet has one wish — to eat more. Now you can have your wish. Recent studies have found that it isn't the amount of food you eat that causes you to gain weight. Rather, it's the type of food. Fat is the main culprit.

GET RID OF THE FAT

Fat composes up to 40% of the calories in the typical daily American diet. Fat is everywhere in our diets. It's hidden in processed foods. It's used to sauté or fry foods. Fat is found in abundance in such good-tasting foods as beef and dairy products (hamburgers and ice cream). Fat is also used as a condiment when we butter our bread, add margarine to our baked potatoes, sauté vegetables in a butter sauce, or top our salads with an oil-based dressing.

Calories from food consist of three categories: protein, simple and complex carbohydrates and fat. Calories are defined as the unit for measuring the energy produced by food when oxidized in the body. We need a percentage of protein, carbohydrates and fat from foods to maintain a healthy diet. But the American diet has shifted to more of a fat-laden diet with the use of more fast foods and processed foods to fit our on-the-go lifestyles.

Various commercial diets try to achieve a total fat consumption of 10-30%, but usually do so through smaller portions. This strategy usually leaves people hungry, and more apt to cravings and binge eating.

WHY FAT MAKES US GAIN WEIGHT

The trouble with dietary fat is that it is very dense compared to carbohydrates or proteins; hence it is less filling. You don't feel as full, so you eat more. A baked potato only has .2 grams of fat and 220 calories, while just one ounce of potato chips has 10 grams of fat and 150 calories. If you wanted to be full, which would you rather eat? Other comparisons include a Hershey candy bar (1.5 ounces) that has 14 grams of fat and 254 calories, one ounce of Cheerios (1.25 cups) which contains 1.8 grams of fat and 111 calories, and a medium apple which has .5 grams of fat and 81 calories.

CUT OUT THE FAT AND EAT TWICE AS MUCH FOOD

Fat has nine calories per gram. Carbohydrates and proteins only have four calories per gram. Thus, fat has over twice the amount of calories per unit compared to other foods. By simply limiting the amount of fat in your diet, you can eat more food. The less fat consumed, the more you can eat. You can be full, eat until you're satisfied and still lose weight.

"Subjects on low-fat diets were able to reach their satiety point by consuming only one-half the calories of those on high-fat diets," according to the May 1983 issue of the *American Journal of Clinical Nutrition* in an article entitled "The Effects of High- and Low-Energy Density Diets on Satiety, Energy Intake, and Eating Time of Obese and Non-obese Subjects," by Duncan, Bacon, and Weinsler. Dean Ornish in his book *Eat More, Weight Less* claims that with his low-fat diet, you can eat more food and lose weight. He further states the body easily converts dietary fat into body fat with little effort.

It only takes 2 1/2 calories to store 100 calories of fat in the body, while it takes 23 calories to convert 100 calories of protein or carbohydrates into body fat. It takes almost 10 times the amount of energy to convert proteins and carbohydrates into body fat. This means you can eat more proteins and carbohydrates, because you burn up more calories in the digestion process.

DIETARY FAT GETS STORED AS FAT

All food must be converted into either fat or sugar for your body to use. Covert Bailey gives a good explanation of this process in his book *Smart Exercise*. He states that the muscles of your body are like an engine that burns two fuels — fat and sugar. When the engine calls for more fuel, it calls on the fat the body has stored. This fat is stored on the hips in women, and in the belly on men. These are our "fuel tanks."

Bailey further states in another analogy that sugar, which is stored in the muscles, functions as kindling, and the fat molecules function as the logs. Both are needed for a good fire. Sugar is used to start the metabolic process that releases energy for the muscles, but fat is required for any long-lasting sustained exercise or muscle action. Bailey contends that getting out of shape means that the muscles lose some of their ability to burn fat due to lack of use for prolonged exercise, and need to be retrained to burn more fat. The best way to do this is through controlled aerobic exercise. Walking is the best aerobic exercise for people who are just beginning an exercise program. It's quick, easy, simple, fun and can be done anywhere.

THE YO-YO SYNDROME

The real secret to losing weight and keeping it off is to control the amount of fat in your diet and to exercise moderately. Just restricting the amount of calories that you eat leaves you craving for more and increases the tendency that most dieters fear — the dreaded "Yo-Yo" syndrome. This is also called the "Feast-or-Famine Cycle."

Most people who have been on a restricted intake diet and then go back to their old habits of eating due to accumulated cravings have experienced this Yo-Yo cycle. It's called the Yo-Yo cycle because every lost pound comes back, usually very quickly. Due to this cycle, many people gain back more weight than they lost on the diet. The explanation for this is tied to human physiology and the way our bodies work.

WHY WE GAIN WEIGHT MORE EASILY TODAY

The availability of an overabundance of food, especially fat, is a relatively new phenomenon. Until the turn of the century, food was a scarce commodity. The main function of most of humanity was to grow and gather food. This wasn't an easy job. Hunting and farming required huge amounts of energy to be expended, sometimes with negligible results. It wasn't until society started to become mechanized, with the advent of the train, motorized farming equipment and refrigeration, that food started to become abundant. This enabled people to move off the farms and establish more of a sedentary, less physically demanding lifestyle. This process has accelerated in the last 40 years.

During this turn-of-the-century period, there were few dietary fats available. Corn-fed, farm-raised animals weren't as prevalent as they are today. Most people ate wild game, which is low in fat (10% to 15%). Farm-raised animals contain up to 30% saturated fat. Milk was hard to come by, and hard to store. Machinery to extract vegetable fats had yet to be invented. The typical diet was over 60% carbohydrates, with fat contributing less than 20%.

The American diet has changed more over the last 100 years than in the previous several centuries. Fat is the most efficient way for the body to store energy. People who could store fat the easiest, and had the most efficient rates of metabolism, were the ones who survived hard times of scarcity, drought or crop failure. Fat people were previously even viewed as attractive and healthy. In fact, in some third-world countries these traits are still cherished.

Our internal physiology has been geared toward storing and saving dietary fat for hard times. When you go on a restricted calorie diet, your body perceives this as a threat of starvation and does many things to compensate. Your appetite and cravings increase, and in extreme cases muscle tissue is sacrificed to preserve stored body fat.

This is why restricted calorie dieters experience the Yo-Yo cycle. When weight is gained back, proportionately more of that weight is stored as fat, as a protection against future lean times.

THE MYTH OF WILL POWER

The myth of will power, that overweight people eat too much, is just that - a myth. Overweight people, in many instances, actually eat less (in calories) than thin people. They probably eat more fat, exercise less and have slower metabolisms. Because of sedentary lifestyles and past failed diets, they have probably been through the Yo-Yo cycle many times. Thus, more of their body weight is made up of fat rather than muscle. Muscle burns more calories, at rest, than fat, while stored fat requires no calories to maintain it on the body.

You will always gain weight back after dieting unless there are changes in eating habits, mostly in the types of food that are eaten. Selecting the right types of food to eat requires little will power, just a bit of education and pre-planning. By decreasing the amount of fat in your diet and increasing your carbohydrate calories, your body won't realize the change. Your body won't react by lowering your metabolism and sacrificing muscle tissue. We probably consume fewer calories than our ancestors did, but much more of it is fat. A simple rule is that if you eat fat, it will make you fat.

EAT, EAT AND EAT SOME MORE TO LOSE WEIGHT

In the book *How to Become Naturally Thin by Eating More*, Jean Antonello lists three ways to stop the feast-or-famine cycle: eat more, eat well, keep eating. Her contention is that if you give your body a continuous supply of food, you break this cycle, and your body will adapt by burning unnecessary stored fuel. Your body will want to burn unnecessary fat.

The key is to eat frequent small meals low in fat — to graze. This will break the feast-or-famine cycle, enabling you to feel full which eliminates cravings, and provide the body with plenty of nutrients so that your metabolism doesn't slow down.

Foods that can be eaten whenever you are hungry include:
- Any and all fruits
- Any and all vegetables (except olives and avocados, both of which are high in fat)
- Grains including whole-grain cereals and breads
- Beans and legumes which provide protein without fat

Foods that can be eaten in moderation include:
- Meats and fish that are low in fat (use smaller portions)
- Non-fat dairy products (not just low-fat; there is a big difference)

Foods that should be avoided include:
- Oils of all kinds (including most salad dressings)
- Meats and fish that are high in fat
- High-fat, and even low-fat dairy products
- Nuts and seeds
- Any processed or fast foods that contain more than 2 or 3 grams of fat per serving
- Most candy and candy bars (hard candy might be acceptable)
- Alcohol

Be cautious of low-fat dairy products. Low-fat milk (listed as 2% fat) actually derives 38% of its calories from fat, or 5 grams of fat per cup. Whole milk and beef are the largest contributors of saturated fats to the American diet.

Fish and chicken, and even vegetables, are often cooked in butter, oil, or margarine which likely defeats any benefit. Steam or microwave vegetables to retain a natural taste without fat. Roasting vegetables is a new technique that is also fat-free.

Meats should be grilled, never fried. Fish can also be grilled, steamed, or poached —- use any cooking method that doesn't need fat. Chicken is low in fat, once the skin is removed (the skin accounts for most of the fat found in chicken). Some fish are high in fat and should be avoided, or eaten in very small portions. These fish include salmon, mackerel and bluefish. Even swordfish and some tunas are high in fat content.

Oils should be avoided because they are nothing more than liquid fat. Any cooking methods that use no or very little oil should be used. Most people would probably lose weight if they did nothing more than eliminate oils and products containing oil from cooking or food preparation. Eating a salad will not be beneficial if you load up on an oil-based salad dressing. Try lemon juice, flavored vinegars, or the fat-free salad dressings now on the market.

COMPLEX CARBOHYDRATES ARE THE KEY

Carbohydrates are great foods because they are low in fat and high in fiber. Fiber gives you that "full" feeling. It takes a good deal more fat-laden foods to give you that same feeling.

There is a difference between complex carbohydrates and simple carbohydrates. Complex carbohydrates include grains, vegetables, and fruits. Simple carbohydrates include sugars, honey, alcohol, and corn syrup (and derivatives).

Simple carbohydrates are absorbed quickly into the body and blood stream and then on to the muscles. This causes less of the stored fat in your body to be burned as fuel. When the body absorbs and burns sugar quickly, blood sugar levels rise and fall rapidly. This will send signals to your body that you need more food. In essence, a rapid decrease in blood sugar levels creates a craving for more sugar.

Having large quantities of refined sugar available is also a recent phenomenon of the American diet. Refined sugar has had the fiber removed. Without the fiber, the warning mechanism that tells your body that you have had enough has been short-circuited. Our bodies haven't adapted, as of yet, to handle this overabundance. Hence, in addition to the dietary fat problem, there is a secondary problem with refined sugar. Sugar is viewed as empty calories with little nutritional value.

CHANGING YOUR TASTES

The next major question is, "How can I stay on a low-fat diet if all the foods I like are high in fat and sugar?" Experts point out that we have no inherent taste for fat. Our taste buds break tastes down into four categories: sweet, sour, salt, bitter. The taste and craving for fatty foods can be broken in a relatively short time by following a low-fat diet.

Fat tends to hide the subtle flavor of foods. After an adjustment time you will once again develop the taste for these subtle flavors. If anyone has ever switched from whole milk to low-fat milk, you know what happens. At first the low-fat milk seems to be watery, but after two or three weeks, when you try to go back to whole milk it almost seems like you are drinking sweet cream.

The experience is similar with salt. At first people on restricted salt diets complain that food has no taste. Two or three weeks later, however, they will tell you that salt, too, masks subtle flavors of food. They can't imagine why anyone would have a salt-shaker at the table as a condiment.

The use of fresh herbs and spices can provide far more intricate tastes on foods than can fat, salt or sugar. It is just a matter of learning how to use these herbs and spices. That is why recipes from our own world-class chef have been included in this book.

THE BIOTECH METHOD - EAT MORE AND LOSE WEIGHT

In this chapter we have learned that by controlling the fat content in our diet, we can eat more food, and weigh less. We will burn more fat than our bodies have stored, and not only will we feel better, but we will look better too. This will not be easy — we are surrounded by fat. The Biotech Plan is unique in that it works permanently, and without deprivation. As an added benefit, those hard-lost pounds rarely return.

The first step in regaining a healthy diet — not the American diet of the last 100 years — is awareness. Once you are aware, you can begin to make the right choices in the foods you eat.

8

EATING YOUR WAY TO A SLIMMER, HEALTHIER BODY

W e've already learned that conventional wisdom, which teaches that the best way to lose weight is by restricting caloric intake, is wrong. In reality, counting calories and limiting food intake is the best way to ensure weight retention and even weight gain.

For proof, you only need to ask any of the estimated 63 million Americans who unsuccessfully attempt to "diet" their way to a perfect shape and weight each year.

One of the reasons conventional diets fail is because they falsely assume that all calories are used equally in the body. This is simply not true. Fat calories are used and stored differently than are carbohydrate calories.

For instance, two Reese's Peanut Butter Cups have about the same caloric value as 1 1/3 cups of cooked rice. But that's about all they have in common.

Granted, the peanut butter cups taste good and are more pleasing to the American palate. The rice, however, is much more likely to be burned up and converted to energy.

Your body does not have a calorie meter, but it does have a "carbo-meter." Carbohydrates activate the hunger switch and stimulate the metabolism. That's why 1-1/3 cups of rice will make you feel more full than the candy. Lots of people could eat 6 peanut butter cups — but how many could eat 4 cups of steamed rice?

WHY TRYING TO CONTROL HUNGER
DOESN'T CONTROL WEIGHT

Hunger is one of the most basic and necessary drives known to man. Faced with starvation, a man will do just about anything, consciously or unconsciously, to obtain food. It's a vast part of the survival instinct.

Any attempt to control hunger, rather than by satisfying it, becomes a matter of fighting your own will to survive. Over the years, man has attempted several schemes designed to suppress this natural urge. These methods generally fall into one of two categories: 1) those that fail and, 2) those that achieve short term success at great risk to health and life.

The methods in the first category usually involve some means of calorie restriction and rely heavily upon will power. Here's the problem. The human mind is goal-driven. It will work tirelessly to obtain the object of our focus. Simply deciding not to eat certain food makes those very foods the center of mental focus. Sooner or later, your will power will lose the war — and usually with a binge.

The methods in the second category attempt to "trick" the body. This can be accomplished though physical intervention, such as purging and diets, which purposely starve the body of important nutrients, or medical intervention, such as drugs and surgery.

Liquid protein diets can cause temporary illness as well as permanently damage the heart, liver and kidneys. Drugs can produce side affects such as nervousness, anxiety, restlessness, irritability, insomnia, dizziness, stomach problems and dry mouth. And surgery, such as stomach stapling and intestinal bypasses, interrupt the proper flow of food causing malabsorption of nutrients and adversely affecting metabolism.

The best way to eliminate nagging hunger and to control weight is to eat the foods your body needs, the foods that turn off your body's natural appetite, the foods that please the taste buds — complex carbohydrates.

EAT YOUR WAY TO A SLIM NEW YOU

A healthy adult needs about 700 grams of carbohydrates per day to meet energy requirements, 20 grams of protein to repair and maintain cells and about 3 grams of fat.

Compare that with the average daily intake of most Americans: approximately 35 grams of fat, 430 grams of carbohydrates and 40 grams of protein. It's no mystery why most Americans struggle with weight control.

Adults need approximately 35 times more carbohydrates for energy than they need protein for growth and they require 800 times more carbohydrates than fat.

By replacing the excess fat and protein in the diet with complex carbohydrates you can win the battle of the bulge — forever. You will be able to eat as much as you want, and there will be no need to count calories or measure food.

In order to kick those calorie-burning ovens into high gear, your body needs to sense that it has access to an unlimited amount of food. Of course it has to be the kind of food that your body needs — complex carbohydrates.

There are seven basic reasons why you must dramatically increase your intake of plant-source carbohydrates in order to lose weight.

CARBOHYDRATE-RICH FOODS ARE LOW IN CALORIES

One gram of carbohydrates contains only 4 calories. One gram of protein contains 5.5 calories and 1 gram of fat contains 9 calories. That means there are more calories in a quarter-pound of fat than there are in a half-pound of carbohydrates.

This fact would be alarming enough if fat calories were utilized in the same way as calories from carbohydrates — but they are not!

CARBOHYDRATES CANNOT BE DIRECTLY ADDED TO FAT STORES

Storing fat calories as fat requires almost no energy. But in order for carbohydrate calories to be deposited, they must first be converted to fat. This conversion process requires 23 calories per 100 calories of carbohydrates.

In other words, of all the calories in a plain baked potato, it would take nearly 1/4 of the fuel in the potato just to convert it to fat. Whereas the tablespoon of butter slathered on top would require no such conversion. It goes straight to the hips or tummy.

CARBOHYDRATES INCREASE METABOLISM

The majority of the carbohydrates we eat are not converted to fat — instead they are broken down into simple sugars. The sugar then stimulates insulin production, and the insulin turns up the production of other hormones. (Mostly norepinephrine and a thyroid hormone called T3.)

These hormones increase the body's metabolism which in turn automatically cranks up the calorie-burning rate. So, to keep our body burning up calories at its maximum level, we need to eat plenty of complex carbohydrates like potatoes, rice and corn.

Limiting carbohydrate intake reverses this process and slows down our metabolism. This makes it even harder to lose those unwanted bulges.

CARBOHYDRATES DECREASE APPETITE

Complex carbohydrates work on the appetite in several important ways. Most plant source carbohydrates are high in fiber which adds bulk to the diet and usually swells in the stomach providing a pleasant sense of fullness.

The sensation of hunger is usually caused by low blood sugar. Plant-source starches and complex sugars help the body maintain a moderate and stable blood sugar level which helps control the urge to binge.

CARBOHYDRATES HAVE HIGHER MASS TO CALORIE RATIO

This fact means that you can eat a much larger volume of carbohydrates than of other foods and get the same number of calories. Consider this: you can consume up to 1600% more volume of carbohydrates than fat for the same amount of calories.

For example, a medium baked potato (approximately one cup) contains about the same number of calories as 1 tablespoon of butter!

So, for the same amount of fat, you can eat up to 16 times as much complex carbohydrates as you can eat in fats. Now, which would you rather have — 1 tablespoon of butter, or 16 baked potatoes? I'll take the baked potatoes topped with fat-free salsa every time! Also, you can consume up to 300% more volume of carbohydrates than animal protein for the same amount of calories. For example, a cup of cooked white rice contains about the same number of calories as 1/3 cup light, water-packed tuna.

COMPLEX CARBOHYDRATES ALWAYS CONTAIN DIETARY FIBER

Aside from adding stomach-filling bulk to your food, dietary fiber has many important health benefits. Significant health research shows that dietary fiber:

- Sucks up cancer-causing substances and drags them away with normal body wastes.
- Binds the fat in cholesterol and helps the body eliminate them. A 1% drop in cholesterol level reduces the risk of heart disease by 2%.
- Decreases the calorie absorption from fats.
- Lowers blood cholesterol levels.
- Stimulates healthy activity of intestines and colon.
- Slows digestion resulting in a higher absorption rate of micronutrients, vitamins and minerals.

One other vital function of fiber is that it increases the efficiency of insulin. The body produces insulin in response to the presence of sugar in the blood. Insulin is required to metabolize blood sugar for utilization by the cells in the body. It also helps in transporting fat to storage in the adipose tissues.

When simple, refined sugars and starches are ingested, insulin levels rise too quickly. Initially there is a sudden burst of energy as the insulin helps "burn up" the sugar in your blood. Soon, however, blood sugar levels drop way below optimum. In response to the perceived need, the brain activates the appetite.

If simple sugars and starches are injected with fat, there is double trouble. Now, in addition to spiking insulin levels and playing havoc with blood sugar, the excess insulin makes you hungry and works to tuck the consumed fat into storage at the same time.

Complex carbohydrates and the accompanying fiber work to stabilize blood sugar and insulin levels, sparing you from this terrible consequence.

CARBOHYDRATES STIMULATE PRODUCTION
OF AN IMPORTANT NEURAL CHEMICAL

Research at the Massachusetts Institute of Technology demonstrated that high carbohydrate consumption increases brain levels of a chemical called seratonin. This neurotransmitter has many physiological and psychological effects on humans. Seratonin triggers a sense of well being. It diminishes hunger, improves the ability to concentrate and enhances sleep.

It is also effective against depression, especially depression experienced from light deprivation and PMS. That explains why people often crave carbohydrate-rich foods during periods of stress and disappointment.

THE SECRET TO EATING YOUR WAY
TO THE PERFECT FIGURE

The secret is: don't limit food quantity, but rather eat foods in proper proportion. Here's how to do it:

1. Use a smaller dinner plate

This may sound a bit contradictory, but it isn't. You should be able to eat until you are full and still achieve and maintain your ideal figure. The important thing is not to eat beyond fullness.

Unfortunately, most Americans have been taught to "clean their plate." So they tend to eat any remaining food on the dish even after their hunger is satisfied.

If you fill and then empty your smaller plate and still feel hungry, go ahead, return for seconds, as long as you continue to eat in the proper proportion.

2. Load your plate using the "clock" method

As you look at your dinner plate, imagine that the face of a clock is painted on it.

Moving clockwise, fill the section of your plate which would be covered by the hour hand moving from 12 o'clock to 1 o'clock with foods that contain between 3 to 6 grams fat per 100 calories. Any foods containing a higher portion of fat should be avoided. These foods can be either entrees or desserts, but remember to keep the fat between 3-6 grams.

Next, fill the section of your plate from 1 o'clock to 3 o'clock with protein foods. This would include lean meats, fish, poultry and no-fat dairy foods.

Finally, fill the rest of your plate, from 3 o'clock to 12 o'clock, with complex carbohydrates. These foods would include fruits, vegetables, whole grains and so on. Refined sugars and simple starches do not belong here.

Rather than counting calories, we'll rely on the volume of foods to guide our selection. The above plan does that quite easily, and is nutritionally sound.

3. Learn to graze

To keep your calorie-burning ovens stoked to their maximum, it is much better to eat many small meals during the day than two or three large meals. In fact, there are some foods that you can eat virtually all day without adversely affecting your

71

waistline. Of course, these must be eaten without fat-based sauces, dressings, dips or toppings.

Here's a partial listing:

Apples	Grapefruit
Bananas	Kidney beans
Beets	Lettuce (all types)
Black beans	Oranges
Broccoli	Onions
Cabbage	Peas
Carrots	Potatoes
Cauliflower	Rice
Celery	Spinach
Corn	Tomatoes
Cucumbers	Zucchini

4. Learn to chew your food completely

Complex carbohydrates require more chewing time than processed foods. Digestion of carbohydrates starts with the introduction of saliva while you chew the food into small pieces with your teeth.

Taking your time and chewing every mouthful 35 to 50 times accomplishes three important tasks. It enhances the flavor of the food — the more broken-down the carbohydrate becomes, the sweeter it becomes. It also allows for more complete absorption of vitamins, minerals and other nutrients in the digestive tract.

Finally, complete chewing slows down food consumption which gives your body more time to react to the fact that you are eating. This results in feeling more satisfaction from a smaller amount of food.

5. Learn to replace the flavor contained in fat

One concern that many people have about avoiding fats is the fear of depriving the taste buds. If that's your worry, there is great news. No- or low-fat doesn't have to be no- or low-flavor.

In fact, a major portion of this book is devoted to proving that low-fat cooking can be every bit as mouth-watering and full of irresistible flavor as its high-fat counterpart.

Once you learn how to use special herbs, spices and fat substitutes in your cooking, you'll see that it's easy to satisfy the palate, fill the tummy and drop the excess pounds all at the same time. Bon appetit!

9

Low-Fat Eating and Vitamin A Reduce Cancer Risks

The typical American diet is anything but healthy. Poor diet and eating habits characterize the day-to-day lifestyles of many, if not most, Americans. This fact alone explains why Americans suffer from some of the most serious diseases in the world.

Poor eating habits, and eating the wrong types of food, expose the body to harmful substances called free radical electrons. Free radicals are not as stable as other electrons. Free radicals are dangerous because they can destroy healthy cells. Recent research demonstrates that free radicals could be a chief cause of changes in the body's cells that lead to cancer. It could well be said that poor eating habits are a large contributing factor to cancer being the most feared disease of Western society.

Many doctors and scientific research teams have shown that eating various types of foods, most notably those high in certain vitamins, enzymes and fiber, can have a dramatic effect on preventing and even helping reverse various cancers. Certain types of vitamins, called antioxidants, and enzymes destroy the free radical cells before they can become cancerous.

DIETARY FAT AND CANCER

There now exists a direct correlation between the amount of fat in your diet and the risk of cancer. In only the last four years, 54 medical and scientific studies have been completed which demonstrate the tie between fat and cancer.[1]

Researchers have linked excess dietary fat intake to cancers of the colon, breast, prostate, pancreas and gastric system, rectum, ovaries, endometrium, larynx, cervix and lungs.[2-7]

RECENT MEDICAL STUDIES CONFIRM THE EFFECTS OF SOME DIETARY PRACTICES ON CANCER

Dietary practice	linked to . . .
Intake of adequate dietary fiber	Reduced risk of rectal polyps and breast, colon, stomach and pancreatic cancer.[8-14]
Intake of adequate fresh fruits and vegetables	Reduced cancer risk of lung, mouth, pharynx, larynx, esophagus, stomach, colon, rectum, bladder and cervix.[15]
Excessive intake of animal fats	Increased risk of prostate cancer.[16]
Intake of foods cooked with oils	Impairment of body's anti-oxidative defense system.[17]
Continued and excessive alcohol consumption	Increased risk of esophageal and pancreatic cancer and increased risk of melanoma.[18-20]
Restricted caloric intake	Lower free-radical activity, increased life span.[21-25]
Intake of caffeine, nicotine	Stimulation of susceptibility to certain cancer conditions.[19]
Excessive intake of iron	Toxic effects of increased oxidative stress.[26]

A study for the American Health Foundation stated that the typical American diet of 40% fat is one of the major risks for cancer, but a low-fat diet in the 20-25% range can reduce the risk.[27]

The Medical Technical Institute in Norway found in a 1994 study that 30% to 60% of all cancers might be caused by dietary factors, most notably the amount of dietary fat. It also stated that fruits and vegetables showed a highly consistent protective effect, indicating that fruit and vegetables may provide general protection against cancer. Five servings of fruit or vegetables are recommended each day to maintain this protective effect.[28]

Researchers at the Center for Disease Control in Atlanta, Georgia stated in 1993 that diet may be an important factor in the cause and prevention of cancer. Experts also linked dietary fat intake to cancers of the breast, colon, rectum, ovaries, endometrium and prostate.[29, 30]

These results have been verified and confirmed by studies done at the University of Nebraska Medical Center, Pennsylvania State University, The Cancer Research Institute and Kanazawa University Hospital.[31-34]

DIETARY FAT, EXCESS WEIGHT AND BREAST CANCER

A large body of medical evidence shows that breast cancer and dietary fat are very closely linked. Researchers draw a direct connection between a diet that has fat levels above 25% and an increased risk of breast cancer. A number of medical studies support this view.

The Karolinska Hospital in Stockholm, Sweden, recommends a low-fat diet for their breast cancer patients, feeling that it is helpful in the prevention and the treatment of cancer. The National Cancer Institute in Bethesda, Maryland, and Michigan State University cite evidence connecting high dietary fat with breast cancer.[35-37]

A 1992 American Health Foundation study demonstrated a 75% reduction in cancer risk using a low-fat diet compared to a high-fat diet. Researchers also determined that total dietary fat should be below 20%, and fiber should be increased to 25-30 grams per day. The Cancer Research Center at the University of Hawaii stated that 10-20% of breast cancer cases could be prevented by decreasing the amount of saturated fat consumed.[38-40]

Columbia University School of Public Health found a possible connection between breast cancer and excess weight in a 1990 study. There was a vast difference between the survival rate of cancer patients on a 20% fat diet compared to the typical American diet containing 35-40% fat. Studies are continuing to determine a more conclusive connection between excess weight and breast cancer.[41]

Researchers at the University of California concluded that a high calorie diet (thus a likelihood for being overweight) is a risk factor for breast cancer. Numerous other studies draw a connection to the intake of dietary fat and breast cancer.[42-51]

DIETARY FAT AND COLON CANCER

Various medical studies indicate that caloric intake and dietary fat content influence colon cancer. One, at the Royal Infirmary in Glasgow, stated emphatically that colon cancer is directly dependent on the amount of dietary fat. The study found that a low-fat diet not only does not produce cancer, but renders colon carcinogens harmless. Simply stated, a low-fat diet prevents cancer, and also destroys carcinogens leading to colon cancer.[52]

The Department of Medicine at St. Luke's Hospital Center in New York concluded in their study that a high-fat diet increases tumors in the colon, and that by restricting calories (fat and/or other calories) colon cancer risk can be reduced.[53]

A direct link between colon cancer and the amount of fiber in the diet was discovered by the University of Toronto. It was found that fiber derived from fruits and vegetables was preferable for its anti-cancer properties.[54]

Further studies indicate that a diet composed of vegetables, grains and fiber resulted in a significant reduction in the risk of colon cancer. It can be shown that there is a link between colon cancer and dietary fat, as well as proof that fruits and vegetables can offer protection against cancer.[54-67]

DIETARY FAT AND PROSTATE CANCER

Only breast cancer has been studied more than cancer of the prostate. As with other cancers, scientists are now becoming more aware of the tremendous role that nutrition plays in preventing prostate cancer.[68, 69]

The Harvard Medical School found that fat consumption was directly related to the risk of advanced prostate cancer. The National Reference Laboratory concluded that prostate cancer could be prevented in up to 35% of the cases by a diet low in fat (under 10%) and high in fiber (40 grams per day).[70, 71]

American men were 26 times more likely to contract prostate cancer than Chinese men. The standard diet in America is very different from that in China, since Americans eat much more fat and much less cereal grains and vegetables.[72]

The Cancer Research Center, the Northern California Cancer Center and the Department of Medicine at the University of Utah all studied prostate cancer. Their conclusion: dietary fat was the strongest risk factor.[73-75]

As this vast body of medical evidence has shown, both for prostate cancer and other cancers as well, a high intake of dietary fat can be a contributing factor for various cancers. Additionally, the increased intake of fruits and vegetables exerts a protective effect on the body, and may reduce the cancer risk by up to 60%.

CANCER AND VITAMIN A

Vitamin A has been shown to have a direct connection to health in mammals. It cleans the cells, and clean cells are high energy cells. It is also important to normal body function. Beta carotene, which is a source of vitamin A, helps eliminate free radicals created during the course of normal cell activity.

There are two types of vitamin A, preformed (usually called retinol), and the provitamin carotenoids (usually called beta carotene). Retinol is found in animal sources like liver, fish, and eggs. Beta carotene is found in plants like yellow fruits, yellow vegetables, and dark-green, leafy vegetables.

You need both forms of vitamin A for healthy eyes and skin, and for the growth and maintenance of teeth, nails, hair, bones, and glands. The most important benefit of beta carotene is as an antioxidant which destroys free radicals. Naturally occurring antioxidants are found in beta carotene, vitamins C and E and the enzyme antioxidants glutathione and catalase (mentioned previously).

The body's own systems defend it from free radical cells thousands of times each day. It performs this task by recombining certain food resources into a substance scientists call "tumor necrosis factor-alpha." It uses this alpha factor to specifically target and dissolve bad cells without killing normal cells or producing side-effects. The scientific and medical data indicates that beta carotene and vitamin A may well be the most important substance for this process of attacking bad cells.

The files at Biotech Research contain 1,207 medical studies and thousands of citations on medical studies performed since 1989, including 183 published studies, discussing the benefits of beta carotene and vitamin A.

In addition to the studies quoted, beta carotene has been used to help reduce free radicals caused by smoking, and for gastritis, certain cancers, DNA damage, Alzheimer's and heart problems. One study found that the dunaliella (algae) form was effective in various cancer conditions.[76-84]

There are literally hundreds of papers demonstrating that vitamin A can suppress the malignancy of cultured cells transformed by radiation, chemicals or viruses. Vitamin A can also delay the development of transplanted tumors and prevent malignancy in animals exposed to various potent carcinogens.[85]

The American Cancer Society and the National Academy of Sciences say that foods that are rich in beta carotene or vitamin A may lower your risk of cancer. The scientific evidence is overwhelming — beta carotene can help reduce or prevent a number of forms of cancer.[86, 87]

A 14-year-long Swiss study, known as the Basel study, determined that there is a direct link between low levels of vitamin A or beta carotene in a person's diet and subsequent death from cancer. Other university studies have demonstrated that beta carotene was toxic to pre-cancer cells, provided protection from certain cancers, and that beta carotene levels were lower in cancer patients. [88-92]

The two most prolific researchers of beta carotene, Drs. Schwartz and Shklar of Harvard University, found that beta carotene begins to inhibit the growth of some human cancer cells within 1-2 hours after eating, and that it could be used to prevent malignancy from cancer.[93, 94]

BENEFITS OF MAINTAINING HIGH LEVELS OF BETA CAROTENE IN THE BODY

- Better health from increased resistance.

- Beneficial for good skin and vision.

- Acts as a powerful antioxidant.

- Helps eliminate free radicals caused by smoking and eating dark roasted foods (coffee) and from radiation therapy.

- Helps keep skin, eyes, and the inner linings of the body more healthy and resistant to infection.

- May help control or prevent mind and memory problems.

- Nutritionally helps prevent certain cancers.

- Helps boosts the immune system.

- Helps in the maintenance and growth of teeth, nails, hair, bones and glands.

Beta carotene helps protect the cells from free-radical damage, and increases the production of natural killer cells that affect some tumor and cancer cell growth.[95, 96]

Natural beta carotene is more powerful than synthetic beta carotene. Eating foods high in beta carotene is an important part of an anti-cancer plan.

Foods that are rich in beta carotene include carrots, asparagus, broccoli, brussel sprouts, cabbage, cantaloupe, cauliflower, spinach, sweet potatoes, and turnips. The most potent source of natural beta carotene is an ocean-grown superfood called dunaliella salina.

AMERICAN DIET LOW IN BETA CAROTENE AND VITAMIN A

Both government and consumer surveys have shown that many Americans are not receiving enough vitamin A and other essential nutrients, even though they may appear to have an adequate diet. Cruciferous vegetables (the cabbage family), such as broccoli and cauliflower, while good sources of beta carotene, are the vegetables that are eaten least.

Beta carotene provides a defense against cancer and its problems. Just by drinking fresh carrot juice daily you will help prevent many of the conditions that cause bad health.

10

VITAMINS AND ENZYMES REDUCE CANCER RISKS

So far, more than 3,000 enzymes have been identified. An enzyme is a complex protein that promotes the speed of a chemical reaction within the body at body temperatures. You can improve your enzyme levels with the proper diet — this will give you more energy and power.

Raw foods that contain high amounts of enzymes are avocados, bananas and mangos. Sprouts are the very highest source of enzymes.

Glutathione peroxidase is a very important enzyme. Made in the body as well as being ingested from food sources, it is an antioxidant that destroys free-radical electrons. Remember that many free radicals come from a high-fat diet. The Chinese Medical Journal concluded that glutathione has an effective antioxidant effect against free radicals.[97]

Researchers in Japan reported that glutathione peroxidase combines with selenium (a non-metallic element that resembles sulfur) to work as a neutralizing factor to help offset some cancers. A follow-up study determined that glutathione and the amino acid L-cysteine (amino acids are the chief components of proteins) was toxic to some tumor cells. The value of glutathione has been proven in other medical studies as well.[98-102]

Glutathione also has been known to have an effect on reducing cholesterol. Various medical studies also point to another enzyme, catalase, as being an important nutritional factor that can offset some types of cancer, as well as being a crucial component of the entire enzyme antioxidant system.[103-105]

VITAMIN C, BIOFLAVONOIDS AND CANCER

Vitamin C is a virtual storehouse of dietary benefits. It acts as an antioxidant, as well as being considered the cornerstone of the vitamin world. Many people think that vitamin C is only a cold and virus remedy. It has uses far beyond that.

Biotech Research has assembled over 150 studies on vitamin C and bioflavonoids. The nutritional power of these food factors cannot be overstated.

Vitamin C and the accompanying bioflavonoids have earned their well-deserved reputation as a nutritional cornerstone. Some experts believe very strongly that high vitamin C intake is a dietary requirement in today's world.

BIOFLAVONOIDS

The bioflavonoids, sometimes called C-complex, were originally called vitamin P by Nobel Laureate discoverer Albert Szent-Gyorgi in 1936. In 1950, biochemist B.L. Oser renamed vitamin P as bioflavonoids.

Bioflavonoids are naturally occurring compounds found primarily in citrus products, but can also be found throughout nature in the plant kingdom. There are three main types: flavones, flavonols and flavonones.

Rutin, citrin and hesperidin are three flavonoids best known for their synergistic effect with vitamin C. Rutin especially is generally accepted as a symptom reliever. It works in combination with vitamin C to prevent persistent bleeding, to care for hemorrhoids, and to keep capillaries from becoming fragile during the aging process.

Most of the general information about vitamin C can also be applied to the bioflavonoids. They are non-toxic and readily absorbed into the bloodstream from the intestinal tract. Any excess is eliminated through perspiration or urination. Bioflavonoid deficiencies are much the same as vitamin C deficiencies. An absence of either vitamin C or bioflavonoids produces the same results — bleeding and bruising are the most common symptoms. Vitamin C and bioflavonoids work together in helping to stabilize many of the body's functions.

Dr. Gyorgyi theorized that the lack of bioflavonoids was partially responsible for health problems in Hungary after World War II. Many of the problems were related to fragile capillaries. Dr. Gyorgyi extracted two different bioflavonoids which were helpful in strengthening the capillaries and prevented bleeding in the tiny blood vessels. The ability of the capillaries to show resiliency is what permits the delicate function of the inner ear. The inner ear controls the functions of hearing and balance.

Research has shown that C-complex is helpful for those with inner ear problems occurring from weak capillaries. One study done in Russia found that children with pollinosis (airborne pollen allergies) experienced relief after taking quercetin, a bioflavonoid.[106]

Another study on quercetin and rutin done in France found that both were effective in preventing the toxicity of oxidized low density lipoproteins (LDL's or cholesterol). This reduces the body's production of free radicals, thereby helping protect the body from cancers.[107]

The lemon has the highest quantity of bioflavonoids. Fifteen to twenty different ones are found in this fruit. Limes, tangerines, grapefruits and oranges also have high amounts but not in as wide a spectrum as lemons. All the different types of bioflavonoids have not yet been catalogued, and some have probably not even been discovered. Bioflavonoids remain an important part of the anti-aging arsenal.

Vitamin C has been called by some experts the single, most effective antioxidant in the human body. This ability enables vitamin C to help correct the nutritional deficiencies responsible for ill health that are caused by free radicals and oxidative stress to the body.

Athletes and sports enthusiasts would benefit by increased amounts of vitamin C. This would help reduce the muscle damage caused by free radicals that are produced as a by-product of physical exertion.[108]

Linus Pauling, of the Linus Pauling Institute, recommends large amounts of vitamin C. Pauling believes that a large intake of vitamin C has no harmful side effects. Vitamin C has been shown to increase longevity in mammals. It cleans the cells, and clean cells are high energy cells.

Vitamin C can add years to human life. It helps slow down the cell damage process from toxins, thus increasing life-span. Some experts think that aging might be controlled by the amount of antioxidants in the body rather than by the physical process of time. Vitamin C and other antioxidants can help keep people feeling and looking younger than their actual age. Aging exposes the body to the greatest threats to health — DNA or cellular damage, heart problems and infections.

The Linus Pauling Institute found in one study that the risk from some cancer can be reduced by up to 80% with the proper amount of vitamin C in the diet. Thirty-three other studies have found that vitamin C prevents various types of cancer.

There are literally hundreds of medical and scientific studies on file in the National Library of Medicine dealing with vitamin C and its nutritional use in various cancers. One study at the University of Missouri concluded in a 1992 report that vitamin C has been associated with cancer prevention.[109]

The Basel study from Switzerland has discovered nutritional relationships between numerous nutrients and various conditions of ill health. The American Journal of Epidemiology reported that vitamin C was associated with a lowered mortality from cancer in general.[110]

One interesting study done at the Massachusetts Institute of Technology discovered that vitamin C was effective as a non-toxic inhibitor of nitrite compounds. Nitrite compounds, such as those found in many foods, have been implicated in a number of health risks.[111] Nitrites are commonly found in most hot dogs, prepared meats and deli-type meat products, as well as being used as a preservative in other types of food products.

Research linked stomach cancer to low levels of vitamin C and high levels of nitrites. It would be prudent for anyone eating foods with nitrites to take vitamin C along with the meal. Be sure to check the ingredient label to determine nitrite content of commonly used foods.

It is important to note that the Leven Hospital in Scotland published a study that documented that vitamin C provided nutritional factors that enabled people with some types of cancer to live almost twice as long as people who did not take vitamin C.[112]

Oranges are the food most associated with vitamin C. They are inexpensive, readily available, and delicious. Other foods rich in vitamin C are citrus fruits, papayas, currants, strawberries, brussel sprouts, green peppers and cantaloupe or honeydew melons.

BENEFITS OF MAINTAINING HIGH LEVELS OF VITAMIN C IN THE BODY

- Vitamin C increases both the number and quality of white blood cells.
- Helps block the cancer-promoting effects of nitrosamines and nitrites.
- Some evidence shows that it can help suppress the growth of human leukemia cells in culture.
- High amounts help boost the body's production of interferon.
- Antioxidant properties.
- Helps retard aging process.
- Leads to better health from increased resistance.
- It's water soluble and helps guard the body against harmful reactions within the cell.
- Helps make capillaries stronger.
- Helps delay capillary fragility of the aging process.
- Helps control bleeding and bruising.
- Helps stabilize inner ear functions.
- Helps restore equilibrium and balance.
- Helps birthing problems in women, bleeding problems, skin problems and other common health concerns.
- Helps combat effects of low vitamin C in smokers.
- Helps eliminate free radicals caused by smoking and eating dark-roasted foods (coffee) and damage from radiation therapy.
- Helps prevent certain cancers.
- May have mild anti-viral effects.
- May help heart problems and ulcers.

VITAMIN E AND CANCER

Vitamin E is an entire family of molecules known as tocopherols. They are broadly classified as either synthetic or natural. While some people maintain that there is no difference between natural and synthetic vitamins, this is not the case with vitamin E. Synthetic vitamin E is very different from natural vitamin E. The natural form is "right-handed" in construction. Synthetic forms of vitamin E are considered "left-handed."

It is important to have an adequate amount of vitamin E, an essential nutrient, in your diet. Vitamin E offers a healthy feeling of accomplishment and well-being.

Vitamin E is rich in sterols, which are potent hormones in the body (hormones are chemicals that originate in a gland and are carried to all parts of the body by the blood). This is why it's reputed to be very invigorating for the procreative and reproductive organs. In fact, vitamin E is so very important for sexual well-being that it has been called the sex vitamin. It also helps reinforce the adrenal glands, bringing increased stamina and athletic endurance.

Researchers at the Research Institute for Medicine and Biology in Japan found that the synthetic vitamin E caused tumors when given to laboratory animals. It can be concluded that synthetic vitamin E provides little if any antioxidant protection from free radicals. For these reasons, only the natural form of vitamin E is recommended for human consumption. This form is found in all foods that are natural sources of vitamin E.[113]

The primary food sources for vitamin E are seed oils and margarines, and shortenings made from these oils. Nuts, seeds, whole grains (the germ), dark leafy green vegetables, eggs and milk are also good sources.

Wheat germ oil contains much more vitamin E than any other oil — 10 IU in a teaspoon. Wheat germ oil is also highly unsaturated and contains large amounts of a powerful fatty acid. Because of this, wheat germ oil has been shown to help strengthen the heart, improve efficiency of muscles, fortify glands, help prevent menopausal symptoms and enhance fertility and virility.

Wheat germ oil is also one of the few oils available that is raw and unrefined. Most clear, golden-colored salad or cooking oils, unless specifically stated otherwise, are refined, bleached, deflavored and deodorized. Some companies use industrial-type solvents in the refining process for their food oils. Cold-pressed or expeller-pressed oils (a natural process that doesn't use solvents) are much superior. This type of oil is reasonably priced and can now be found in most supermarkets and grocery stores.

Be careful about the type of oil used for cooking. A study done at the National Nutrition Institute in Italy found that heated unsaturated oils produce noticeable reductions in the body's antioxidant defense system.[114]

The Surgery Department at the University of Cincinnati College of Medicine found that vitamin E was useful in various conditions of ill health, namely certain cancers, immune system and heart problems. They concluded that nutritional therapy using supplements is an old idea now becoming increasingly important.[115]

A 1991 study done in Helsinki, Finland, found that people with low levels of vitamin E increased their risk of getting cancer by 1 1/2 times over people who had a higher intake of vitamin E.[116]

The Chinese Academy of Medical Sciences found that vitamin E can reduce some cancer risk by as much as 33%. The Cancer Biology Laboratory in 1990 found that vitamin E — when given in combination with selenium, vitamin A and other substances — could reduce the presence of some cancerous tumors by up to 91.7%.[117, 118]

Russian researchers found that vitamin E helped to protect the liver and red blood cells in leukemia cases. Laboratory tests have shown that deficiencies of vitamin E result in a higher incidence of some cancers.[119, 120]

University of Kansas researchers concluded that dietary levels of vitamins C and E have been associated with cancer prevention and to a lesser extent with therapeutic enhancement of cancer treatment. A Harvard study states that vitamin E appears to prevent tumor formation by stimulating a potent immune response to selectively destroy tumor cells as they begin to develop into recognizable microscopic foci of carcinoma. The Dartmouth Medical School demonstrated that vitamin C and E have a clear preventive effect on tumor formation.[121-123]

At particular risk for cancer and infection are the elderly and young children. Researchers in Tokushima, Japan, found that extra amounts of vitamin A and E stimulated the immune system, and were especially important in helping prevent lung infections (viral and bronchitis-type problems) and some cancers.[124]

There are over 184 studies on vitamin E in the files of Biotech Research. Vitamin E has a proven antioxidant power in many conditions of ill health. Vitamin E has been studied for its nutritional value in various types of cancer, as well as in chemical, toxic substance and radiation-caused problems.

BENEFITS OF MAINTAINING HIGH LEVELS OF VITAMIN E IN THE BODY

- Better health from increased resistance.
- Vitamin E appears to have anti-blood-clotting effects.
- Adds to selenium's cancer-fighting antioxidant effects.
- Helps slow down the aging process.
- May improve circulation.
- Helps relieve leg pain when walking.
- Vitamin E helps protects the good fatty acids from free radical attack.
- Helps improve the efficiency of the heart.
- Studies have shown that vitamin E helps protect against damage from environmental pollutants and cigarette smoke.
- Antioxidant properties help eliminate free radicals caused by smoking and eating dark-roasted foods (coffee) and free-radical damage from radiation therapy.

FOODS HIGH IN VITAMIN E

- Sunflower seeds or oil
- Sesame seeds or oil
- Almonds or oil
- Canola, soy or corn oils
- Wheat germ
- Whole grain products
- Liver
- Dried beans
- Dark green leafy vegetables

COENZYME Q10 AND CANCER

Coenzyme Q10 has been found to increase energy levels, enhance free radical antioxidant activity, possibly improve heart muscle power and help cellular energy. Q10 is the most important enzyme for the body's energy levels.

Rich food sources of Q10 are beef heart, mackerel, sardines and other meats and fish. Cereals, brans, peanuts, dark leafy green vegetables and soybeans are good sources as well.

Much of Q10's benefits apparently come from its antioxidant status. The Department of Food Science and Technology of the University of California at Davis found that Q10 was an effective free radical destroyer. It was also shown that Q10 decreased free radical activity in the liver, kidney and heart.[125]

As mentioned earlier, free radicals are damaged cells in the body that can become cancerous. Thus, coenzyme Q10's antioxidant activity can reduce the likelihood of free radicals mutating further into tumors or cancer cells.

As the body ages, liver production of coenzyme Q10 declines. That is one reason everyone needs to consider foods that are nutritionally dense in Q10 levels. One study found that Q10 can decline by up to 80% in the course of normal aging.

Studies done at Huddings Hospital in Sweden found that the protein content, as well as the Q10 content of the brain decreases continuously with age. It was also noted that Q10 levels in the brain change radically in Alzheimer's patients, thereby implying that Q10 intake could play a part in this disease.[126, 127]

Coenzyme Q10 levels in the body begin to decline at about 20 years of age. Before that, it remains relatively high. This explains why energy levels sometimes drop when a person reaches the early 20s. By age 30, the body can be up to 11% deficient. At 40, when fatigue may become more common, Q10 levels are around 14% short. Once these deficiency levels rise above 30%, the likelihood of other health problems increases.[128]

NUTRITIONAL BENEFITS OF COENZYME Q10

- Can help increase energy.
- Can improve exercise tolerance.
- Can help combat age-related declines in bodily defense systems.
- Helps resist harmful bodily peroxides (free radicals).
- Helps stimulate the immune system.
- Helps protect mitochondrial membranes with its antioxidant properties.
- Helps to promote better feelings of well-being.

BEST FOOD SOURCES FOR
FREE-RADICAL-FIGHTING NUTRIENTS

VITAMIN A
Beef Liver
Dandelion Greens
Sweet Potatoes
Dried Apricot
Pumpkin
Cooked Spinach
Collards
Dried Red Peppers
Raw Watercress
Cooked Kale

CALCIUM
Swiss Cheese
Milk, whole or skim
Yogurt, low-fat
Tofu
Turnip Greens
Sardines, in oil
Salmon, canned, pink
Kale
Broccoli
Navy Beans

VITAMIN C
Currants
Strawberries (frozen)
Brussel Sprouts
Orange Juice (fresh)
Lemon Juice
Papaya
Grapefruit Juice
Green Peppers
Cantaloupe
Collards

MAGNESIUM
Cod Steak
Lima Beans
Black-eyed Peas
Garbanzo Beans
Whole Milk
Granola
Oatmeal
Avocado
Dried Figs
Broccoli (cooked)

VITAMIN E
Sweet Potato
Walnuts
Asparagus
Sunflower Seeds
Almonds
Hazelnuts
Brussel Sprouts
Broccoli
Wheat Germ
Apple (medium)

ZINC
Beef Chuck
White Meat Chicken
Salmon
Raw Eastern Oyster
Split Peas
Chicken Eggs
Whole Milk
American Cheese
Bran Flakes
Brown Rice

11

LOW-FAT EATING REDUCES HEART DISEASE RISKS

Research has now confirmed that proper eating habits can have a dramatic effect on preventing and even reversing various diseases, among them the several different types of cardiomyopathies (chronic disorders of the heart muscle) and other heart problems.

Dozens of medical studies point to proper nutrition as a key factor linking diet to hypertension, atherosclerosis, elevated cholesterol levels, ischemic heart disease and cardiovascular disease in general.

Experts have found that eating the proper foods, and maintaining an ideal weight, plays a crucial part in preventing heart disease and in recovering from already existing disease conditions.

For every square inch of unneeded fat, the body must produce an additional 700 miles of small blood vessels called capillaries. Thus, the heart must work harder to keep blood pressure at optimum levels as additional capillaries are added to the body, mostly in excess fat deposits.

People who are overweight usually do not exercise sufficiently. This creates a doubly dangerous situation — the heart must work harder to make blood flow through extra capillaries, and the heart is likely at a lower range of muscle tone due to lack of exercise.

Put more simply, a fat, flabby heart has a hard time coping with the additional burdens that may be placed upon it. People with under-exercised but overworked hearts are at a greater risk of heart problems or even early death. Excess weight is not just a matter of appearance, it is actually a life-or-death situation.

The Biotech Plan accomplishes what has been impossible before this — a way to easily lose weight and exercise the heart. And a way to do all of this while having fun!

DIETARY FAT AND HEART DISEASE

Numerous studies point to the role that excess dietary fat plays in various heart problems, such as ischemic heart disease (temporary deficiency of blood to the heart), atherosclerosis (a form of hardening of the arteries), hypertension (high blood pressure) and elevated cholesterol levels.[129]

The VA Medical Center in San Francisco found that the risk of dying from a heart-related condition could be lowered by as much as 20% simply by reducing fat in the diet, which would then lower blood cholesterol.[130]

Pennsylvania State University stated that excessive dietary fat is associated with a number of disorders, including obesity and heart disease. The reason for high fat consumption was due to its palatability. In simple language, fat tastes good.[131]

The University of Toronto was a little bolder and stated that research points to childhood as the critical period when these dietary patterns are initiated. The desire for regular physical exercise is also established while young. The findings document that if you make lifestyle changes, even late in life, there will be a marked effect on your physical condition.[132]

As far as cholesterol problems, an interesting medical study was done by the Connor research team at Oregon Health Sciences University. Their conclusion was that diet therapy for lowering cholesterol should be the main treatment, and that drug therapies should be added to the diet program only as needed.[133]

The emphasis on diet was confirmed by numerous studies including those done at Boston University and the Iwate Medical University in Japan.[134,135]

Atherosclerosis, a form of hardening of the arteries, has been studied extensively. Researchers at the Bowman Gray School of Medicine found that limiting the use of saturated fats and using only polyunsaturated fats in the diet reduced the risk of this heart condition. The study demonstrated that use of polyunsaturates in childhood would have a beneficial effect, and likely reduce the risk of heart problems later in life.[136]

Other research showing the same benefit of reduced fat consumption has been conducted at Stanford University and the Department of Medicine at Oregon Health Sciences University.[137,138]

High blood pressure has also been studied and a connection was found to high fat consumption as well.[139]

Without doubt, the most interesting study was conducted at Loma Linda University in California, where researchers tried to determine if eating walnuts had a beneficial impact. They found that when 20% of the diet was replaced with walnuts, cholesterol readings were reduced by as much as 16.3% in only four weeks. So, to lower your cholesterol, go ahead and enjoy yourself — eat a handful of chewy, delicious walnuts! But go easy on them — they still contain fat (meaning weight gain).[140]

Many other medical studies have found a relationship between excess fat in the diet and heart problems, namely high blood pressure and cardiovascular disease.[141-143]

By the way, evidence is mounting that the use of margarine may not be as beneficial as once thought. A research team at the University of Athens, Greece, found that cooking with margarine increased the risk of coronary heart disease.[144] You might want to try cooking with a no-fat cooking spray in a non-stick pan, or use a scant drop of a polyunsaturated oil.

HEART DISEASE AND FOOD ENZYMES

The glutathione peroxidase enzyme is very important, as we've already discussed in Chapter 4 on reducing cancer risk. This enzyme is also valuable for its use in reducing the risk of various heart diseases.

Researchers determined that glutathione, as well as catalase (another enzyme) levels were lower in cardiomyopathy (a chronic heart disorder), and concluded that this heart problem may be brought on as we age and also by changes in the immune system.[145]

Glutathione is a proven antioxidant that reduces lipid peroxide (cholesterol) and free radical levels. The Chinese Medical Journal associated dilated cardiomyopathy to free radical damage. It was concluded that glutathione is effective in its antioxidant effect against free radicals.[146]

Catalase is another enzyme that not only plays a role in preventing cancer but heart disease as well. The University of Tennessee found that catalase helped to prevent the narrowing of the blood vessels in the lungs, injury to the small capillaries, and an excessive buildup of tissue fluid in the lungs.[147]

Most Americans suffer from low enzyme levels. This situation can be improved or eliminated entirely, helping to provide increased levels of energy and power. The Biotech low-fat eating plan incorporates the use of raw vegetables and fruits which help to remedy this unhealthy condition.

Raw foods that contain high amounts of enzymes are avocados, bananas and mangos. Sprouts are the very highest source of enzymes.

VITAMIN A-RICH FOODS AND HEART PROBLEMS

Beta carotene, a form of vitamin A, has received favorable publicity regarding its nutritional uses in helping prevent many types of cancer. Beta carotene has also been found to be helpful in correcting nutritional factors associated with various heart problems.[148]

The Upjohn Research Clinic in Michigan found that low amounts of beta carotene (15 mg) daily increased the amount of high density lipids (HDLs) in the bloodstream. HDLs are commonly known as "good cholesterol" since they help scavenge cholesterol deposits from the arteries.[149]

The Cardiology Department at the University of Edinburgh found that the higher the level of carotene in the bloodstream, the lower the risk of heart problems. They concluded that those people with a high incidence of heart-related problems could possibly benefit from a diet rich in natural antioxidants.[150]

Researchers at the University of California discovered much the same, finding that beta carotene helped cause a decrease in cholesterol and a similar decrease in free radicals.[151]

These findings and others have been verified at such institutions as the Arteriosclerosis Prevention Clinic at the University of Kansas, the University of Kuopio in Finland, Skodsborg Hospital in Denmark and various institutions throughout Russia.[152-158]

Synthetic beta carotene does not provide the benefits that natural beta carotene does, as demonstrated in the studies done at Harvard University.

As discussed previously, the standard American diet is low in beta carotene and vitamin A, but this is a rather simple condition to remedy by increasing the intake of carotene-type foods. Foods rich in beta carotene are carrots, asparagus, broccoli, brussel sprouts, cabbage, cantaloupe, cauliflower, spinach, sweet potatoes, and turnips. Interestingly, you can eat most of these foods in unlimited amounts on the Biotech Plan.

VITAMIN C AND HEART PROBLEMS

Like many other nutrients, vitamin C has a host of uses in the human body. It is also important in a good anti-heart disease program.

Medical studies done in 1991 show that vitamin C and bioflavonoids help with certain heart problems and are powerful antioxidants.[159,160]

Problems with blood vessels, especially of the eyes, and lowering of blood pressure have been helped with vitamin C and bioflavonoids.

Experts at the Harvard School of Public Health found that vitamin C helps protect against heart problems caused by low density lipids. Vitamin C does this by helping destroy free radicals before they can attack healthy cells. Vitamin C also increases the body's resistance to ion oxidation.[161]

The Nutrition Laboratory of the U.S. Department of Agriculture states that vitamin C helps to lower cholesterol as well as systolic and pulse pressure in people with hypertension.[162]

University of Kansas Medical Center researchers came to the same conclusion in their study that vitamin C reduces susceptibility of low density lipids to oxidation. The conclusion was that a vitamin C supplement could have a great impact on heart problems.[163]

In his book *Nutritional Influences on Illness*, Dr. Melvyn Werbach reported that cholesterol levels dropped 41 points in six weeks after taking daily doses of vitamin C (1000 mgs). Just this one heart tip could save the lives of thousands of Americans every year.

These are a few of the many scientific studies done since 1989 researching the use of vitamin C and its role in helping various heart problems.

Most people know that oranges are full of vitamin C. They are inexpensive, readily available, and delicious. Other foods rich in vitamin C are citrus fruits, papayas, currants, strawberries, brussel sprouts, green peppers, and cantaloupe or honeydew melons.

VITAMIN E AND HEART DISEASE

The Arteriosclerosis Prevention Clinic at the University of Kansas Medical Center noted that recent research suggests nutritional antioxidants could have a great impact in the prevention of heart problems. Many other medical studies discuss the nutritional use for vitamin E in people with heart problems.[164]

The University of Cincinnati College of Medicine found that vitamin E was useful in various heart conditions.[165]

Researchers at the Ciba-Geigy Laboratory in New Jersey found that a vitamin E supplement helps protect the heart against injury from oxygen deprivation, which is commonly called a "heart attack."[166]

Three studies determined that is it possible to predict whether a person would die of a heart-related ailment by measuring the amount of vitamin E in the bloodstream. The University of Berne in Switzerland found that using this vitamin E method in addition to blood pressure readings, they had 87% accuracy rate in predicting heart problems.[167,168]

The researchers at Hoffman-La Roche Laboratory in Basel, Switzerland, (home of the famous Basel Study) determined that by using the vitamin E method and including cholesterol levels, heart problems could be predicted with a 94% accuracy rate.[169]

Norman Bethune University found that deficiency of vitamin E could lead to Keshan Disease, a serious heart problem, which could be prevented by increasing vitamin E intake.[170,171]

Numerous researchers have looked at coronary heart problems and the nutritional relationship with vitamin E. Edinburgh University researchers concluded in two studies that some people with a high incidence of heart problems could benefit from natural antioxidants like vitamin E. Similar studies from Hoffman-La Roche and the Geriatric Clinic in Switzerland produced similar results.[172,173,158]

In animal testing, vitamin E helps prevent artery clogging due to plaque buildup. Without vitamin E, an LDL particle contains only eight to ten antioxidant molecules. These few molecules can only do so much. A higher blood level of vitamin E means fewer free radicals.

Vitamin E is found in seed oils and margarines, and shortenings made from these oils. Nuts, seeds, whole grains (the germ), dark leafy green vegetables, eggs and milk are also good sources.

Wheat germ oil, high in vitamin E content, has also been shown to help strengthen the heart. As discussed in Chapter 3, it is also a very good oil to use. Please use it sparingly. Since it is not low-fat, a little will go a long way.

HEALTHY HEART BENEFITS FROM MAINTAINING HIGH LEVELS OF VITAMIN E IN THE BODY

- Vitamin E appears to have anti-blood-clotting effects.
- Helps improve circulation.
- Helps improve the efficiency of the heart.

CHROMIUM

Chromium is an essential nutrient. Deficiencies can lead to possible diabetic symptoms, glucose intolerance, nerve disorders, impaired growth, elevated blood cholesterol, deposits, decreased lifespan, decreased fertility and other health problems. Chromium, also called glucose tolerance factor (GTF), first achieved attention for its importance in the 1950s. Be sure that any supplement you use is the organic Trivalent form.[174-179]

Chromium and magnesium have been used to help heart integrity. Chromium, in particular, has been shown to help protect against certain heart problems, high cholesterol and high blood pressure.[180-182]

A number of studies have shown that nations with the lowest levels of chromium consumption had higher amounts of adverse cardiovascular conditions. These same nations also had the highest levels of refined carbohydrate intake (sugar). The Food and Drug Administration and the Food and Nutrition Board, in tentative Recommended Daily Allowances, suggests daily amounts of chromium between 50-200 micrograms.

Chromium has been shown to be important in maintaining normal lipid (fat) and carbohydrate metabolism and reducing harmful buildup in arteries. Studies at Mercy Hospital in San Diego showed that chromium picolinate (the most effective form of chromium) is effective in lowering fat levels in the blood.[183,184]

When autopsies were done on individuals who died of heart attacks, biopsies of their major blood vessels often failed to show any chromium present. Several researchers have found that a chromium supplement helped to lower blood sugar and cholesterol.

The average diet of millions of Americans is chromium-poor because of our taste for refined foods. Chromium levels also dramatically decline with age. Proper amounts of chromium are essential for good health.[175]

Chromium picolinate, a specific form of chromium, is the best form of chromium to use as a diet supplement and has received attention in programs that reduce body fat and increase muscle mass.

Food sources for chromium include brown rice, cheese, meat, whole grains, dried beans, chicken, corn, calves' liver, mushrooms, and potatoes.

COENZYME Q10

A coenzyme is the protein portion of a vitamin. Of all the nutritional food factors, coenzyme Q10 shines as the star when it comes to protecting and nourishing the heart. The greatest amount of coenzyme Q10 is found in the heart and liver. Q10 also helps with high blood pressure problems. Some of these benefits were noted by scientists in as few as nine days.[185-195]

Biopsies done on the heart tissue of individuals with certain heart problems have revealed deficiencies in Q10. Scientific studies indicated that patients afflicted with varying heart problems had lower than normal levels of Q10 in their myocardia (heart muscle) or muscle tissue mitochondria (organelles found within the cell that produce energy).[196,197]

The Karolinska Institute in Stockholm, Sweden, determined that patients with heart problems lost Q10 at a faster rate than hypertensive patients, and that this low ratio of Q10 indicated an increased risk.[198]

The Institute of Cardiology in Rome found that Q10 was deficient in the heart tissue of patients, and after receiving a supplement, 47% of the patients experienced a regression of adverse symptoms.[199]

Q10 also decreased episodes of angina by as much as 53%, and patients significantly increased their ability to do a treadmill test when given 150 mgs. daily for four weeks.

Scientists found improvements in 82% of the patients that were given a daily dose of Q10 (100mg). For individuals with high blood pressure, 91% of those treated with 60 mgs daily experienced a 10% reduction in blood pressure rates.

Japanese researchers at the Showa University School of Pharmaceutical Sciences found that smaller amounts of Q10 were synthesized in conditions of heart ischemia (deficiency of blood flow). Other Japanese researchers at Kobe University found that Q10 helped restore a more regular heart rhythm within 10 minutes.[200]

DOCTORS USE Q10 WITH HEART CONDITIONS

Coenzyme Q10 has been used nutritionally by doctors for certain heart conditions at the Methodist Hospital in Indianapolis and the Institute for Biomedical Research at the University of Texas.

Doctors and researchers found that 91% of their heart patients showed improvement within thirty days after taking coenzyme Q10 as a diet supplement.[198]

The American Journal of Cardiology published research that coenzyme Q10 was helpful in relieving painful heart conditions. Research at the Free University in Brussels demonstrated that Q10 helped boost the performance of the heart, even where there were severe cardiac conditions. Research at the University of Texas found a three-year survival rate for congestive heart failure increased from 25% to 75% with the use of Q10. And they also found, along with the Center for Adult Diseases in Japan, that Q10 can help lower high blood pressure.

The Hiroshima University School of Medicine showed that nutritional therapy using Q10 and free radicals can play an important role in preventing myocardial injury.[201]

Rich food sources of Q10 are beef heart, mackerel, sardines and other meats and fish. Cereals, brans, peanuts, dark leafy green vegetables, and soybeans are good sources as well.

12

Walking: The Best Weight Loss Exercise

Exercise is a key to staying fit and healthy. It is often frustrating for some overweight people to eat less, sometimes much less, than their slimmer counterparts and still gain weight. This happens because overweight people have lost some of their ability to burn fat.

As explained previously, the body burns two fuels - fat and sugar. Sugar is the fuel that is used first. Only after the sugar that's stored in the body starts to get depleted is fat used as fuel. Fat, when used as fuel, requires oxygen to burn. This is the essence of aerobic exercise - perform some activity that uses oxygen to burn stored fat.

Exercise should be strenuous enough to require stored fat to be burned, but not hard enough to make you short of breath.

THE FAT-BURNING EXERCISE TEST

A good gauge of proper aerobic activity is this - you should be able to exercise and still talk without becoming short of breath. In this way, you're burning up the maximum amount of fat with the exercise, and pumping maximum amounts of oxygen through your body.

Exercise that makes you short of breath is called anaerobic. During anaerobic exercise, little if any fat is burned, sugar is only burned half-way and lactic acid builds up in the muscle. Lactic acid is what creates muscle soreness after you exercise.

WALKING - THE BEST FAT-BURNING EXERCISE

The best way to lose fat might be a brisk walk, or the dance-type aerobics exercise class at the health club. Walking is the most natural function of the human body. We use almost every muscle in our bodies when we walk. The skeletal and muscular systems come together in the human body to form a perfect walking machine. There are literally dozens of health and emotional benefits derived from walking.

Walking will help you to:
- Maintain your weight at the proper level.
- Burn off excess fat.
- Decrease your appetite.
- Lower the amount of fat (cholesterol levels) in the blood.

Walking can also help to:
- Decrease the risk of heart attack.
- Increase the supply of oxygen in the blood.
- Improve and control blood circulation.
- Increase "good" cholesterol (high-density lipids or HDL's).
- Improve the elasticity of blood vessels.

Walking has been shown to:
- Reduce tension.
- Keep bones strong.
- Relieve some discomforts of arthritis.
- Help muscle tone and improve your looks.

In short, walking can help you to stay fit for life, more so than any other form of exercise. Other more strenuous forms of exercise will probably not keep you as fit overall, likely because these short bursts of strenuous activity will not be sustained. Walking is also a safe sport, not having the injuries common to more strenuous activities.

Oxygen, the most vital ingredient to our survival, cannot be stored in the body. Without oxygen, we die in about five minutes. Walking will help increase the supply of oxygen in the blood stream, and hence, to every muscle, organ, tissue and cell in the body. This increased supply of oxygen will improve the efficiency and functions of all the body's systems.

Walking is the exercise that is most efficient in producing physical fitness. Good fitness helps keep the body free of disease. Walking makes us healthy without the risk of injury or over-straining the body. The shape, structure and flexibility of the spine means that we are better suited for walking than sitting, standing, or running.

Walking is also the "bridge" to help us get back into shape for other sports or physical activities that might be more taxing on the body.

WALKING IS FUN AND EASY TO DO

Walking is inexpensive, can be done by anyone, can be done almost anywhere, and can be done by the entire family. You have probably noticed the walking "explosion" as it has grown in popularity over the last few years. When the weather is nice, walkers are seen all over the neighborhood or at the local walking track. During inclement weather, walkers are found at the shopping malls and health clubs.

Walking can be done in a variety of speeds and styles to fit every fitness level.

Covert Bailey in his book, *Smart Exercise,* compares the enzymes that burn fat molecules to a labor union. (Enzymes are complex organic substances that promote the speed of various chemical reactions in the body). This union goes on strike whenever there is not enough oxygen. Muscles, as you exercise, start begging for more fuel because they use it quickly. Whenever a muscle contracts, there is demand for fuel. The fat-burning union is happy as long as it is paid with enough oxygen. But it strikes as soon as it looks like there might be a shortage. Meanwhile, the sugar-burning union has more faith in management and keeps working.

Bailey says the secret is to make the fat-burning union work as hard as possible without going on strike. If this work can be sustained for long periods of time, eventually more fat-burning workers will need to be hired. The opposite is also true - if you are a coach potato who gets little or no exercise, fat-burning workers will be laid-off.

When these fat-burning union workers are laid-off, it's easy for an overweight person to gain weight while eating less than a thin person. Lean muscle tissue has a faster metabolism rate than fat tissue. This just compounds the situation and frustrates the overweight person even more.

Overweight people can turn this whole scenario around with moderate exercise. During exercise, fat tissue is lost, and you gain muscle tissue by adding more fat-burning enzymes. Exercise will increase your metabolism, and you will burn off calories faster. This wonderful benefit of an increased metabolism also carries over to those times when you're not exercising. Yes, it's possible to increase your body's fat-burning power just by adding a walking program to your lifestyle.

WALKING SOLVES MANY DIETING PROBLEMS

By adding more fat-burning enzymes and building more muscle tissue, you can burn more calories without lowering the "set point" on your internal thermostat.

The "set point" theory of weight management is the theory that every person has an individual "thermostat." This thermostat controls the quantity of food that your body demands. There is speculation that the amount of fat that will be stored in the body is also controlled in this way. Overweight people often have a hard time losing weight because this thermostat calls for more calories and creates a craving.

Care should be taken not to lower this "set point" on the thermostat by fasting or by strenuous anaerobic exercise. Both could actually cause your body to conserve calories and fat by slowing your metabolism. Scientists have a word for this: "homeostasis."

Homeostasis is the tendency for the body to keep things constant or in a similar state, making dieting by traditional means difficult.

WALKING AND COMPLEX CARBOHYDRATES ARE THE KEY

The key is to fool the body by eating more calories so the body won't lower the "set point." But be careful not to eat fat — your body will try to store fat right back where you just burned it up. Eating carbohydrates quiets the body's cravings. More calories need to be burned to turn carbohydrates into fat than to turn dietary fat into fat. Burning fat to build muscle, such as that which occurs during walking or aerobics, raises the "set point," because muscle burns more calories than fat.

WHY CALORIE COUNTING DOESN'T WORK

On a restricted calorie diet, you may stop losing weight as your body slows your metabolism. The more times you go on a diet, the lower and lower the "set point" becomes as your body readjusts due to homeostasis. This is what causes you to gain back more weight than you lost, even if you just go back to eating the same amount of food you did before you started the restricted-calorie diet. Some studies have found that when these cycles of dieting take place, it takes twice as long to lose weight, and weight is gained back even faster.

This explains why dieting, as it has been practiced over the last 20 or 30 years, is so frustrating. Fighting all of the various defenses that the body uses to keep in a state of equilibrium is very hard. The cravings, the lowering of the metabolism, the set point, the burning of sugar, the Yo-Yo cycle, the laying off of the fat-burning union workers (as in Bailey's analogy) all work against losing weight. No wonder most dieters can't lose weight and keep it off. Making a conventional diet work against all of these defenses is an impossible mission.

Jean Antonello in her book, *How to Be Naturally Thin by Eating More*, states that a conventional diet with a strenuous exercise program creates a physiological catastrophe — a severe famine. Once the muscle and liver stores of glycogen (sugar) are used up, and the body still needs more energy in a hurry (anaerobic exercise), the next recourse of the body is to break down protein and burn muscle, not fat.

Soon, undesirable symptoms set in. Fatigue, muscle weakness, excessive hunger and restlessness are common when muscle tissue is burned.

You must listen to the signals from your body and heed them, as your body has important information on what it needs if you just tune in.

This is why you experience cravings for certain foods. If you are trying to lose weight, it is wise to ignore any cravings for fat until your weight range is reached. You should reach instead for any of the low-fat foods that you can eat anytime. Look at the chart of these foods found in Appendix B of this book.

SPEED UP THE FAT-BURNING PROCESS

We've learned about the body's tendency to protect itself from weight loss and fat loss. We learned that the body can be fooled by eating less fat and more carbohydrates, which along with aerobic exercise, will cause body fat stores to be burned. By converting fat tissue to muscle tissue we can raise the set point of our metabolisms, therefore burning more fat. Sometimes, building muscle tissue and losing fat tissue is a long process. Is there any way to add more of the fat-burning enzymes to speed up this weight loss process?

Fitness experts maintain that wind sprints are the fastest way to improve fitness and increase the number of fat-burning enzymes. Exercise to the point of being slightly out of breath, and then return to normal walking. Sprint 2 or 3 times during a 30-minute walk to the point where you are slightly out of breath. For an overweight person who is out of shape, sprinting can be replaced by a brisk walk. For a person in moderately good shape, a wind sprint might mean a quick jog. For a person in good shape it might involve running.

The fat-burning union workers will be fine when walking is the extent of the exercise. When jogging takes place every once in a while, more fat-burning union workers are needed. These workers don't really want to strike all the time. After all, picket lines are hard work too. It's time to hire a few more fat-burning workers for those times when a little jogging takes place.

MAKING EXERCISE FUN

But why should I have to do all of this exercise now, you might ask? You never had to do this when you were young, and you stayed in great shape. Well, when you were young and in shape, it wasn't called exercise — it was called fun. Children are in constant motion. It isn't called aerobic exercise. It's called playing. Throwing the frisbee, hide-and-seek in the back yard, running to see your friends in the neighborhood (remember when you didn't have a car), chasing lightning bugs, riding your bike to the store or school — all of the wonderful, fun ways to burn calories.

As we age, there is a natural tendency to slow down. We must learn to fight this tendency. After about age 30, the heart begins to lose its ability to pump blood at the rate of 6% to 8% per decade. Lungs lose some of their resilience, and muscle mass is lost at the rate of 3% to 4% a decade. If you are inactive, you will age faster.

Therefore, we must make a conscious decision to exercise, walk, or somehow get physical motion into our lives. If walking and exercise are unappealing, we need to look around and discover other ways.

Use the stairs instead of the elevator, walk to the corner store, rent a parking space a couple of blocks away at work, make sure the laundry room is a floor away, park in the back lot at the mall. Those are just a few examples.

The beauty of the Biotech Plan is that you are free to design your own program around your likes and dislikes. After all, the program that you design will likely be the one that you can stay with and enjoy for life.

WARMING UP FIRST BURNS MORE FAT

Remember — it's important to warm up before any exercise. A well-known theory states that oxygen doesn't detach itself from hemoglobin easily in a cold muscle. If you have ever experienced shortness of breath when just beginning to walk or jog, but later (at the same speed) had no problem, then you probably had a brush with this physiological occurrence.

As muscle temperature rises, oxygen breaks away from hemoglobin more completely and quickly. If you didn't warm up you were probably experiencing anaerobic exercise. So, if you warm up first, you'll be able to burn more fat without experiencing anaerobic exercise and the accompanying shortness of breath.

Exercise also helps to lower blood pressure. Athletes typically have very low blood pressure, more red blood cells, and more plasma content in the blood than non-active people. Raymond Kurzweil states in his book, *The 10% Solution for a Healthy Diet*, that fat causes blood to thicken. He says that this is why you feel groggy after eating a meal rich in fat. This fat-laden blood has difficulty passing through the smaller capillaries, thus depriving the brain of oxygen.

WALKING FIGHTS HARDENING OF THE ARTERIES

Kurzweil makes the strong claim that 90% of all Americans have a serious and potentially fatal disease —atherosclerosis. Atherosclerosis is a form of hardening of the arteries. He says that the analogy of atherosclerosis as a grease buildup in pipes is not accurate. It is reversed. The plaque (grease) is hard, and the pipe (artery) is soft. The study sited for this 90% figure was done in 1955 on American soldiers killed in Korea. Autopsies gave evidence of atherosclerosis in 77% of a relatively young subject group — 22 year-old soldiers. If there is that much evidence of this disease in young soldiers, then it follows that it exists in out-of-shape older people as well.

Kurzweil states in his book that atherosclerosis is a progressive disease with a buildup of plaque in the wall of the arteries. This narrows the passageways and leaves less room for blood. When these passageways are constricted to 70% of their original size, there is a danger of blood clots forming. These blood clots sometimes cause heart attacks and strokes. Kurzwell states further that this disease is symptom-free, and that 60% of the people who die of a sudden heart attack never had any warning.

Fat in the diet is the major source of this plaque on the artery walls. This has been proved by many studies in countries that still have low-fat diets. Many third world nations have diets that are low in fat because the people can't afford fatty processed foods or farm-raised beef. As the living standards are raised, many of those people begin to experience the same fat-caused health problems as Americans.

Fitness experts contend that this effect can be counteracted by exercise. Exercise will add plasma to the blood. Plasma is watery and flows easily through the arteries. The added red blood cells will help deliver oxygen during fat-burning aerobic exercises.

The increased muscle mass gained by exercise will form more capillaries which will enable the blood to thin out. Studies demonstrate that aerobic exercise will raise the levels of HDL (high density lipoprotein), or good cholesterol, which can help clean up freshly-deposited plaque in the arteries before it has a chance to harden.

GET FIT FOR A LONG LIFE

The physical deterioration associated with old age is not normal to the human species, but is the result of a high-fat diet. It is basically the culmination of decades of consuming toxic fat. I can still remember seeing news clips of Jack LaLanne swimming across the San Francisco bay towing a rowboat filled with reporters on his 65th birthday celebration. He knew the benefits of lifelong activity, and it served him well.

Low-fat eating is easy and delicious. Exercise will have you looking fit in no time, and you'll be so excited by the way you look. So break out of those old routines and ruts and become a new you!

13

How To Turn
Your Body Into A
Fat-Burning Machine

Little in life stimulates more envy than watching a skinny person eat like there's no tomorrow — every day — without gaining an ounce! Why is it that some people eat like a horse and look like a fox and others can eat like a mouse and put on pounds like a cow?

A small portion of the answer is related to heredity — some people are just born with a hyperfast metabolism. However, metabolic rate is much more controllable than most people realize. A very significant portion of our metabolic rate is controlled by what we eat. (That aspect of metabolism is thoroughly discussed in Chapter 2.)

But, there is a much more important factor governing the speed at which our bodies burn the fuel we eat. That factor is the ratio of body fat to lean muscle mass.

HOW OUR PERCENTAGE OF BODY FAT AFFECTS WEIGHT CONTROL

One pound of body fat requires only 2 calories per day to maintain itself. On the other hand, a pound of muscle tissue consumes many times more fuel — even at rest.

Depending on the developmental level, each pound of muscle burns from 30 to 50 calories per day just to maintain itself. A body that has 40 pounds of muscle will burn a minimum of 750 to 2,000 calories in a 24-hour period — just to stay alive.

That means that the calorie requirements for two people who have the same weight, height, and body frame but who have different percentages of body fat can vary dramatically.

For example:

	Person A	Person B
Height:	5'5"	5'5"
Weight:	134 lbs.	134 lbs.
Frame:	Medium	Medium
Percent fat:	31% (41.3 lbs.)	25% (34.1 lbs.)
Percent muscle:	33% (44.5 lbs.)	41% (54.9 lbs.)
Calories to maintain fat @ 2 Cal/lb.	83 Calories	68 Calories
Calories to maintain muscle	1335 Calories	2086 Calories
Total Maintenance	1418 Calories	2154 Calories

Person B can eat 600 calories per day more than Person A — without gaining weight! Plus, Person A would gain weight on a 1600 calorie per day diet and Person B would lose about 1/2 pound per week, not counting any loss from exercise.

In other words, every pound of fat that you replace with a pound of muscle will require 15 to 25 times as much food — just to exist!

To estimate your percentage of body fat, refer to Tables 1 and 2.

TABLE 1
WOMEN'S PERCENT FAT ESTIMATION CHART

HEIGHT IN INCHES

HIP MEASUREMENT IN INCHES	56	57	58	59	60	61	62	63	64	65	66	67	68	69	70	71	72	73
32	20	19	19	18	17	16	16	15	15	14	14	13	13	12	12	11	10	10
33	22	22	21	20	19	19	18	17	17	16	16	15	15	14	14	13	12	12
34	24	24	23	22	21	21	20	19	19	19	18	17	17	16	16	15	14	14
35	26	26	25	24	24	23	22	21	21	21	20	19	19	18	18	17	16	16
36	29	28	27	26	26	25	24	23	23	23	22	21	21	20	20	19	18	18
37	31	30	29	29	28	27	26	25	25	25	24	24	23	22	22	21	20	20
38	33	32	31	31	30	29	28	28	27	27	26	26	25	24	24	23	23	22
39	35	34	34	33	32	31	30	30	30	29	28	28	27	26	26	25	25	24
40	37	37	36	35	34	33	33	32	32	31	30	30	29	28	28	27	27	26
41	39	39	38	37	36	35	35	34	34	33	32	32	31	30	30	29	29	28
42	42	41	40	39	38	38	37	36	36	35	34	34	33	33	32	31	31	30
43	44	43	42	41	41	40	39	38	38	37	37	36	35	35	34	33	33	32

☐ OPTIMUM RANGE

WOMEN: To estimate your percent of body fat, follow the row corresponding to your hip measurement (in inches) to the column which lists your height (in inches). The shaded area represents the optimum percent fat ranges for women. If a more accurate determination is desired, consult with a fitness center in your area.

TABLE 2
MEN'S PERCENT FAT ESTIMATION CHART

WEIGHT IN POUNDS

WAIST (in.)	120	125	130	135	140	145	150	155	160	165	170	175	180	185	190	195	200	205	210	215	220	225	230	235	240	245	250	255	260
27	7	6	5	5	5	5	5	4	—	—	—	—	—	—	—	—	—	—	—	—	—	—	—	—	—	—	—	—	—
28	9	8	7	7	6	6	6	6	5	5	—	—	—	—	—	—	—	—	—	—	—	—	—	—	—	—	—	—	—
29	11	10	9	9	8	8	7	7	6	6	5	5	—	—	—	—	—	—	—	—	—	—	—	—	—	—	—	—	—
30	13	12	11	11	10	10	9	8	8	8	7	6	6	5	5	—	—	—	—	—	—	—	—	—	—	—	—	—	—
31	15	14	13	12	11	11	11	10	10	10	9	8	8	6	6	5	5	—	—	—	—	—	—	—	—	—	—	—	—
32	18	17	16	15	14	13	13	12	12	12	11	9	8	8	6	6	5	5	—	—	—	—	—	—	—	—	—	—	—
33	21	20	19	17	17	15	15	15	14	14	13	11	9	9	8	6	6	5	5	—	—	—	—	—	—	—	—	—	—
34	23	23	21	20	20	17	17	17	16	16	15	13	11	11	9	8	8	6	6	5	5	—	—	—	—	—	—	—	—
35	27	26	24	23	22	20	19	19	18	18	17	15	13	13	11	10	9	8	8	6	6	5	5	—	—	—	—	—	—
36	30	30	28	25	25	23	23	23	21	21	19	17	15	15	13	11	11	9	9	8	7	6	6	5	5	—	—	—	—
37	34	34	31	28	29	25	26	26	23	23	21	19	17	17	15	14	13	11	11	9	9	8	7	6	6	5	5	5	—
38	40	38	35	32	31	28	28	28	25	26	23	21	19	18	17	16	15	14	13	11	10	9	8	7	7	6	6	5	5
39	—	40	40	36	35	32	31	29	28	28	25	23	21	19	18	17	16	15	14	13	11	10	9	8	8	7	7	6	6
40	—	—	40	40	40	36	35	34	31	31	28	25	23	21	19	18	17	16	15	14	13	11	10	9	9	8	8	7	7
41	—	—	—	41	41	41	40	39	38	36	35	34	31	31	28	25	23	21	20	19	18	17	16	15	14	13	10	9	8
42	—	—	—	—	42	—	—	42	42	40	39	38	35	34	33	31	31	29	28	27	25	24	23	22	20	19	18	17	15
43	—	—	—	—	—	—	—	—	—	42	41	40	38	37	35	34	33	31	29	28	27	25	24	23	22	21	20	19	17
44	—	—	—	—	—	—	—	—	—	—	—	40	39	38	38	37	35	34	33	31	29	28	26	25	24	23	22	21	19
45	—	—	—	—	—	—	—	—	—	—	—	—	—	40	40	39	38	37	35	34	33	31	29	28	27	26	25	24	23
46	—	—	—	—	—	—	—	—	—	—	—	—	—	—	—	40	40	40	38	38	36	34	33	31	31	29	28	27	25
47	—	—	—	—	—	—	—	—	—	—	—	—	—	—	—	—	40	40	39	39	38	37	35	34	33	31	31	29	28
48	—	—	—	—	—	—	—	—	—	—	—	—	—	—	—	—	—	—	40	40	40	39	38	37	35	34	33	31	31
49	—	—	—	—	—	—	—	—	—	—	—	—	—	—	—	—	—	—	—	—	41	40	38	37	36	35	33	33	32
50	—	—	—	—	—	—	—	—	—	—	—	—	—	—	—	—	—	—	—	—	40	—	40	39	37	37	36	36	35

WAIST MEASUREMENT IN INCHES

☐ OPTIMUM RANGE

MEN: To estimate your percent of body fat, follow the row corresponding to your waist measurement (in inches) to the column which most closely matches your weight (in pounds). The shaded area represents the optimum fat ranges for men. If a more accurate determination is desired, consult with a fitness center in your area.

THE COMPLETE FAT-BURNING EXERCISE PROGRAM

There are two types of exercise — aerobic and anaerobic. Aerobic exercise burns fat immediately, as the exercise is performed. Anaerobic exercise, however, burns almost no fat during the exercise session. It is this fact that made fitness experts believe that anaerobic exercise was not beneficial for weight loss.

It is now clear that both types of exercise aid in the elimination of excess body fat and both are necessary for total fitness and health. But there are many significant differences.

Aerobic exercise is any activity that gets the respiration and pulse within 60% to 80% of its maximum rate for a minimum of 10 minutes at a time. There are many advantages to aerobic exercise, in addition to burning fat. It helps lower heart rate and blood pressure, increases hemoglobin levels and the capacity to combat stress, and it builds cardiovascular fitness.

Anaerobic is a short-term (10 to 60 seconds), high intensity, low repetition workout that builds muscle mass. Several recent studies demonstrate the important role developed muscle mass plays in burning calories and fat.

One study compared a group that dieted and did 15 minutes of aerobic exercise plus 15 minutes of weight training 3 times a week with a group that dieted and did 30 minutes of aerobic exercise only. The group that did weight training *and* aerobic exercise lost twice as much weight and 2 1/2 times as much fat as the aerobic group.

To really appreciate the value of an exercise program that emphasizes aerobic and anaerobic activity, study Tables 3 and 4 and the accompanying chart. The fact is, the more exercise you do, the more fit you become. The more fit you become, the more exercise you can perform and the more calories and fat you can burn. Therefore, a regular program of aerobic and anaerobic exercise will turn your body into a lean, fat-burning machine.

As long as you stay in your range and avoid losing your breath, your aerobic workout can be accomplished by biking, swimming, walking, jogging, running or other similar activity. And, the more of your body that you involve, the more calories you will burn.

The next section of this chapter will show you how to have an effective, no-special-equipment-needed anaerobic workout. These exercises help you build muscle and strength.

CHART 1

How a program of aerobic and anaerobic exercise increases caloric requirements. This chart demonstrates the increased calorie need created by a program of aerobic and anaerobic exercise as weight loss is accomplished. The data for this chart appears in Tables 3 and 4 below. Note: a weight loss program without exercise actually lowers daily caloric requirements.

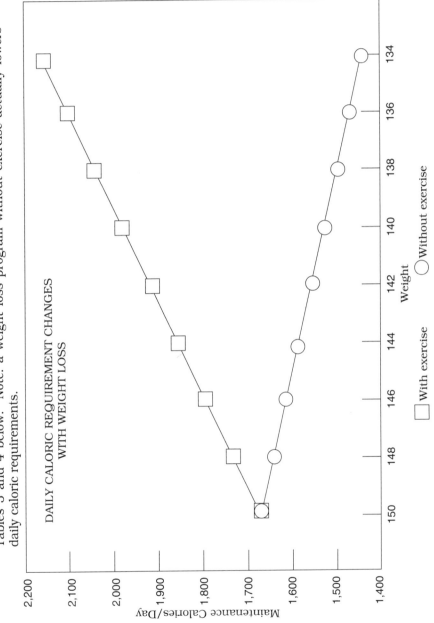

DAILY CALORIC REQUIREMENT CHANGES
WITH WEIGHT LOSS

TABLE 3
DECREASE IN MAINTENANCE CALORIES IN WEIGHT LOSS PROGRAM WITHOUT EXERCISE PROGRAM

	Weight	% Muscle	Pounds Muscle	Maint. Calories Per lb.	Maint. Calories Muscle	% Fat	Pounds Fat	Maint. Calories Fat	Total Maint. Calories
Start	150	0.350	52.5	30	1575	0.350	52.5	105.0	1680
	148	0.348	51.5	30	1545	0.345	51.1	102.2	1647
	146	0.346	50.5	30	1515	0.340	49.7	99.4	1614
	144	0.344	49.5	30	1485	0.335	48.3	96.6	1582
	142	0.342	48.5	30	1455	0.330	46.9	93.8	1549
	140	0.339	47.5	30	1425	0.325	45.5	91.0	1516
	138	0.337	46.5	30	1395	0.320	44.1	88.2	1483
	136	0.335	45.5	30	1365	0.314	42.7	85.4	1450
End	134	0.332	44.5	30	1335	0.308	41.3	82.6	1418

TABLE 4
INCREASE IN MAINTENANCE CALORIES IN WEIGHT LOSS PROGRAM WITH ANAEROBIC AND AEROBIC EXERCISE PROGRAM

	Weight	% Muscle	Pounds Muscle	Maint. Calories Per lb.	Maint. Calories Muscle	% Fat	Pounds Fat	Maint. Calories Fat	Total Maint. Calories
Start	150	0.350	52.5	30	1575	0.350	52.5	105.0	1680
	148	0.357	52.8	31	1637	0.339	50.2	100.4	1737
	146	0.364	53.1	32	1699	0.328	47.9	95.8	1795
	144	0.371	53.4	33	1762	0.317	45.6	91.2	1853
	142	0.378	53.7	34	1826	0.305	43.3	86.6	1912
	140	0.386	54.0	35	1890	0.293	41.0	82.0	1972
	138	0.393	54.3	36	1955	0.280	38.7	77.4	2032
	136	0.401	54.6	37	2020	0.268	36.4	72.8	2093
End	134	0.410	54.9	38	2086	0.254	34.1	68.2	2154

THE BIOTECH EASY-EXERCISE METHOD

The following movements work over 90% of the muscles in the body. They are designed to work the six major muscle groups — legs, chest, back, shoulders, waist and obliques.

The instructions are really quite simple. Exercise each muscle group for 5-10 minutes, 3 or 4 times per week. The entire program takes as little as 25 minutes.

For instance, the leg exercises consist of easy or hard lunges, step ups and squats. You could do lunges for 2 minutes, step ups for 2 minutes and squats for 2 minutes. Your leg work has taken only 6 minutes and you are now finished with leg exercises for the day. Then, go on to the chest, back, shoulder, waist and oblique exercises.

For each movement, work up to 30 repetitions. When you can do 30 reps, move on to the next degree of difficulty exercise for that muscle group. For example, when you can do 30 easy pushups, move on to the hard pushups.

It is best to alternate days that you exercise, with a day of rest in between each workout day. Following this plan, you will notice obvious improvement in only 3 weeks or less.

If you experience any sudden pain, tearing or popping of a muscle, discontinue exercising immediately and rest for a few days or consult a sports physician.

If you experience any soreness after exercising, you can try the following remedies to help relieve the discomfort:

1. Increase rest days to 2 days between each workout day.

2. Stretch slowly before you begin your workout session. Also try to stretch slowly to relieve any soreness.

3. Use heat, such as a hot bath, shower or whirlpool.

4. Gently massage the muscle. You can have a friend or family member do this for you, or you might visit a local massage or massotherapist.

For the one arm row exercises, fill the suitcase with books or other items that weigh anywhere from 20-30 pounds.

An interesting sidenote: Taunya, one of my clients photographed for the exercises in this book, is the mother of 4 children. She looks good and is in excellent physical condition. If she can do it, so can you. Let's get started...

LEGS
This group of exercises works the quadricep (thigh), hamstring and gluteus maximus and minimus (derriere) muscles.

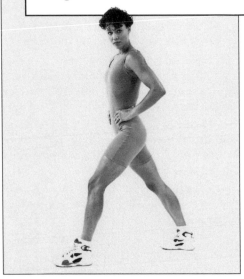

Easy lunge (begin)

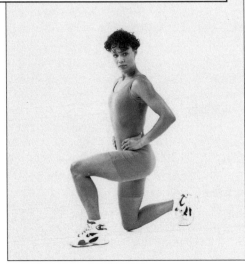

Easy lunge (end)
(Switch and do other leg also.)

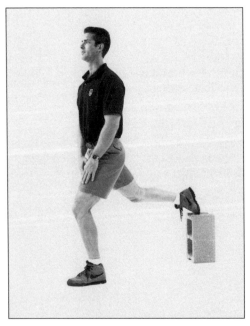

Hard Lunge (begin)

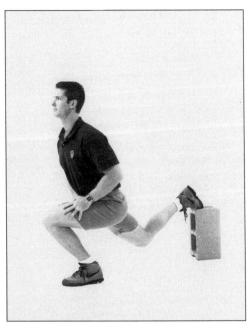

Hard lunge (end)
(Switch and do other leg also.)

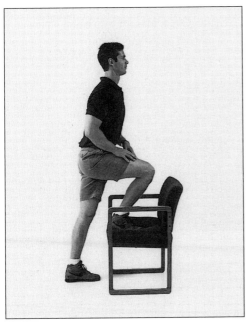

Chair stepup (begin)

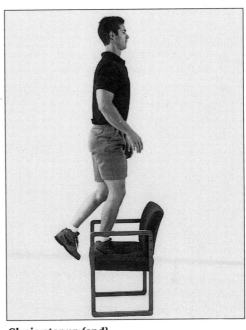

Chair stepup (end)
(Switch and do other leg also.)

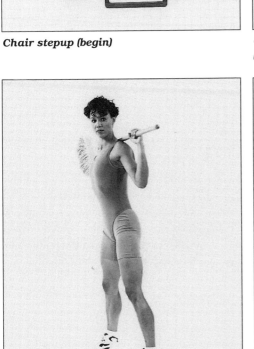

Broomstick squat (begin)

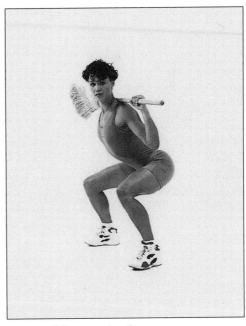

Broomstick squat (end)

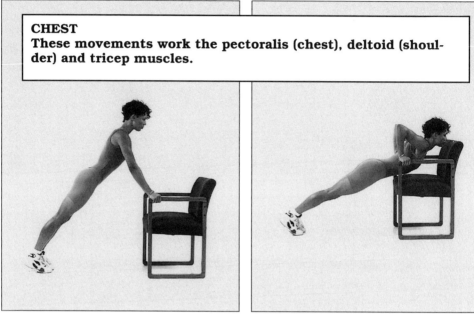

CHEST
These movements work the pectoralis (chest), deltoid (shoulder) and tricep muscles.

Easy pushup (begin)

Easy pushup (end)

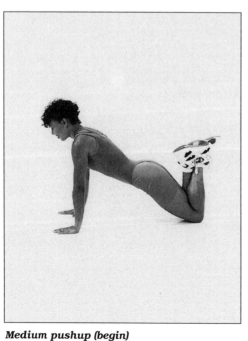

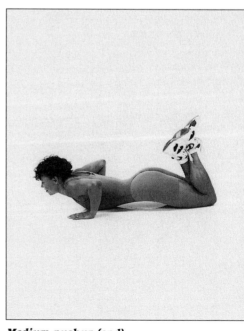

Medium pushup (begin)

Medium pushup (end)

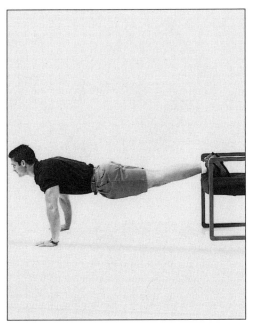
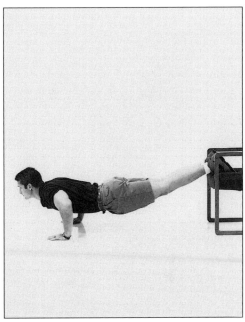

Hard pushup (begin)   *Hard pushup (end)*

BACK
These exercises work the latissimus dorsi (back), trapezius, rhomboid and bicep muscles.

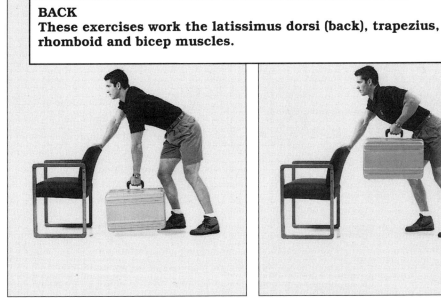

One arm row (begin)   *One arm row (end)*
(Switch and do with other arm also.)

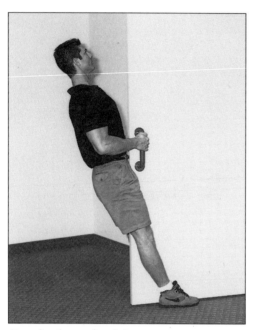

Door knob row (begin)

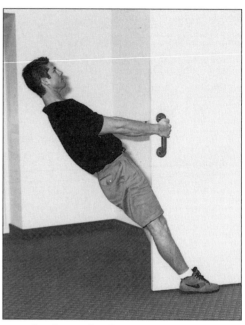

Door knob row (end)

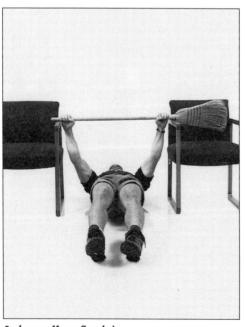

Lying pull up (begin)

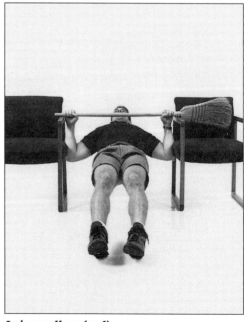

Lying pull up (end)

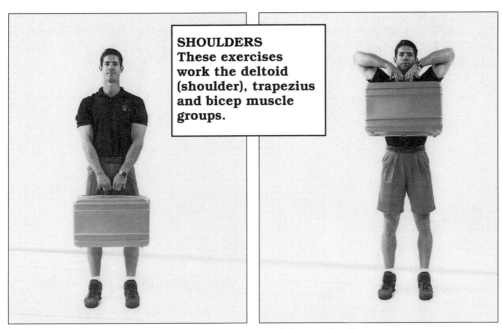

SHOULDERS
These exercises
work the deltoid
(shoulder), trapezius
and bicep muscle
groups.

Upright row (begin)

Upright row (end)

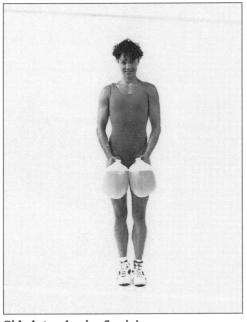

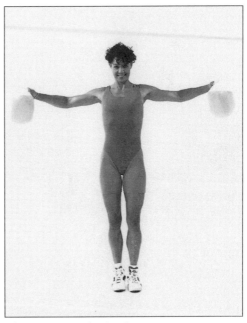

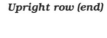

Side lateral raise (begin)

Side lateral raise (end)

113

WAIST
These movements work the various abdominal and oblique muscle groups.

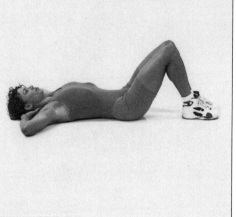

Crunch (begin)

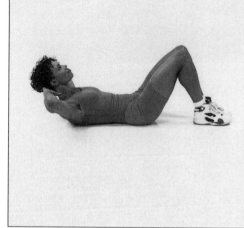

Crunch (end)

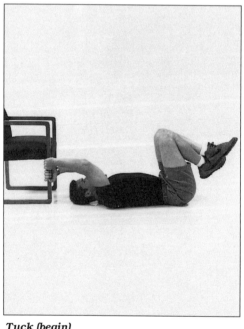

Tuck (begin)

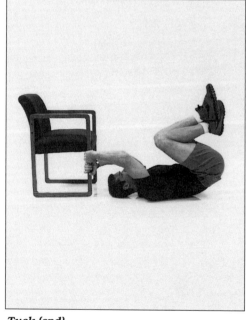

Tuck (end)

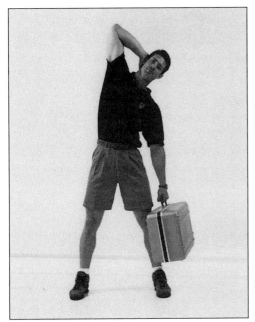

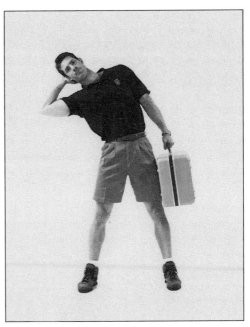

Side bend (begin)

Side bend (end)
(Switch and do other side also.)

CHEF EDWARD'S GOURMET LOW-FAT RECIPES

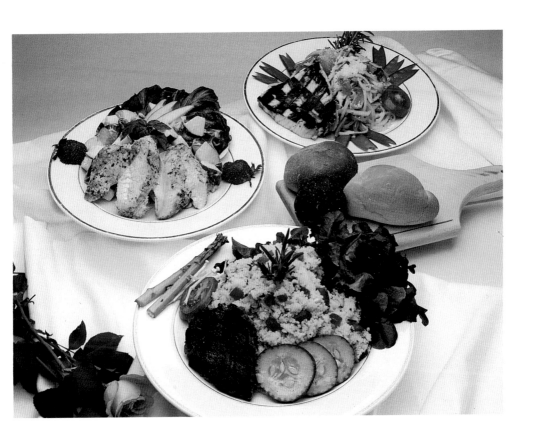

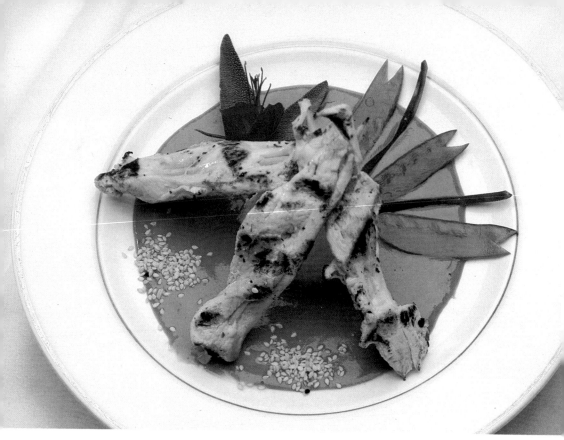

Chicken Satay appetizer (see page 137)

Grilled Sesame Halibut (see page 155)

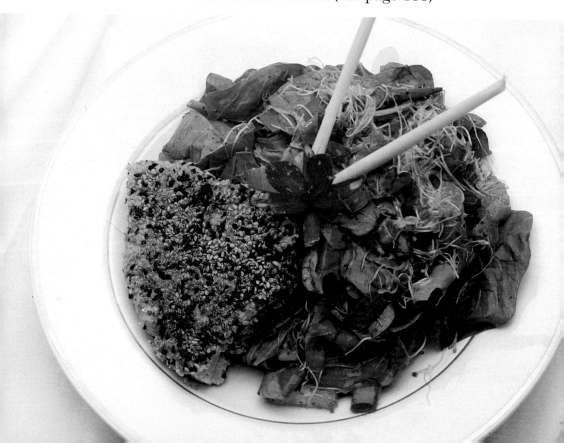

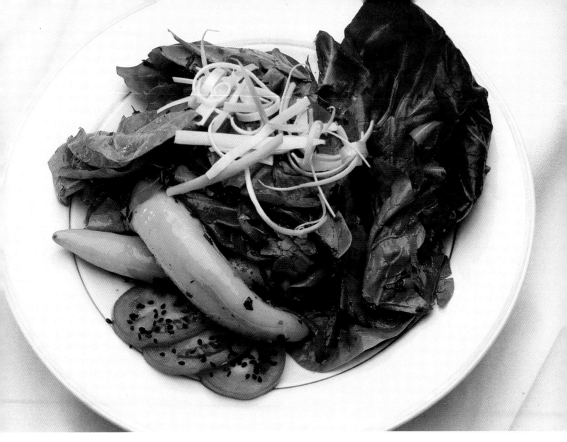

Banana Peppers and Spinach salad (see page 141)

Chicken Waldorf salad (see page 139)

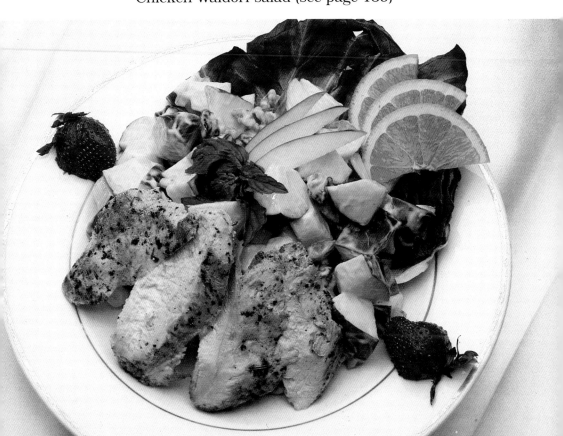

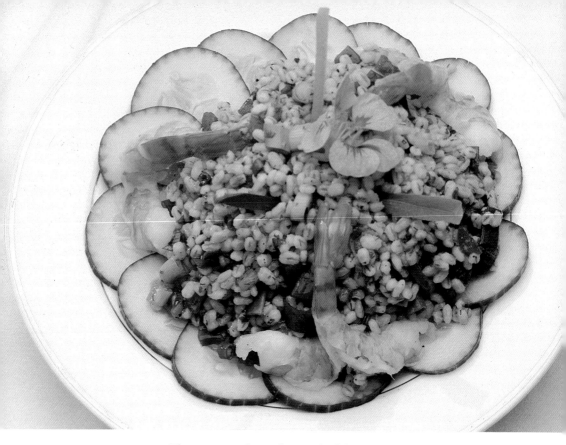

Shrimp and Barley salad (see page 141)

Grilled Roma Tomatoes (see page 141)

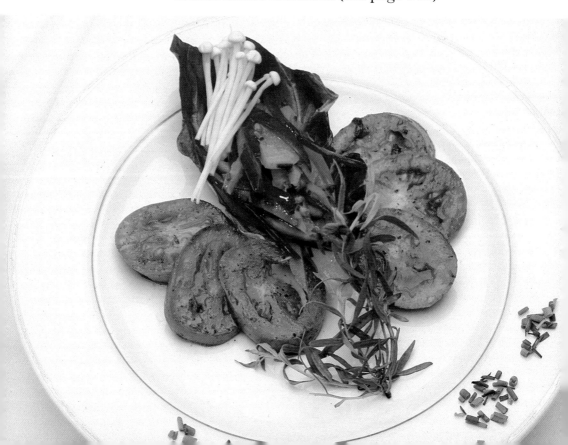

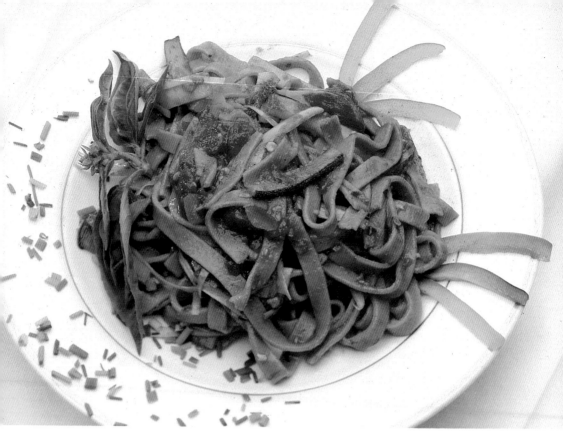

Tomato Fettuccine (see page 162)

Charbroiled Chicken with Pineapple Chutney (see page 153)

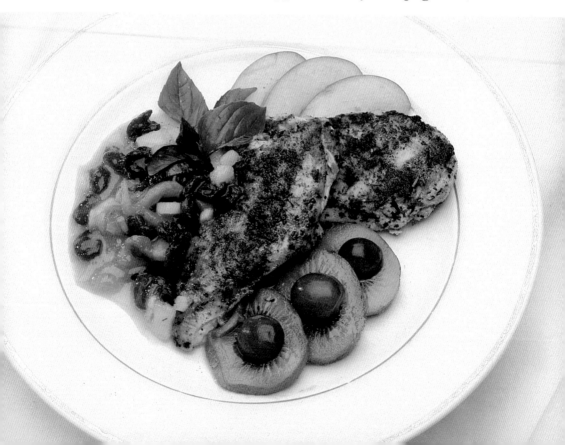

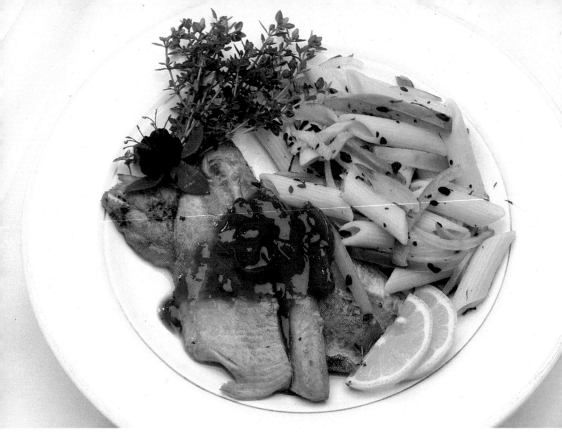

North Carolina Grilled Trout (see page 158)

Breast Of Chicken Palombo (see page 154)

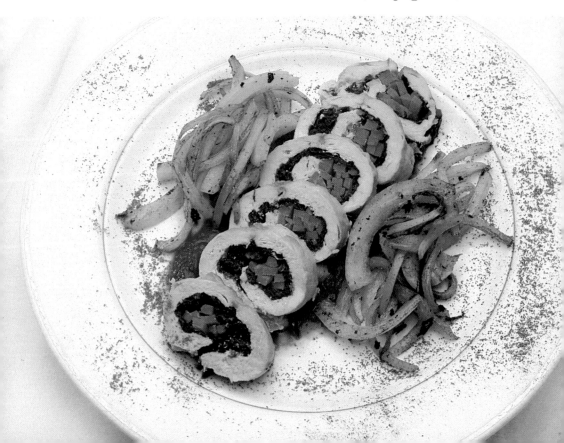

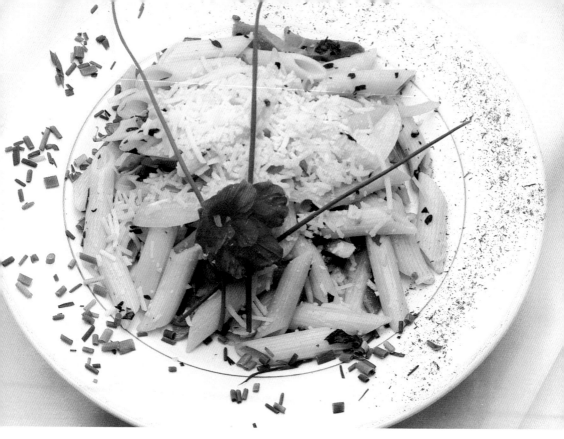

Penna Pasta, Ham and Snow Peas (see page 161)

Grilled Tenderloin of Beef (see page 149)

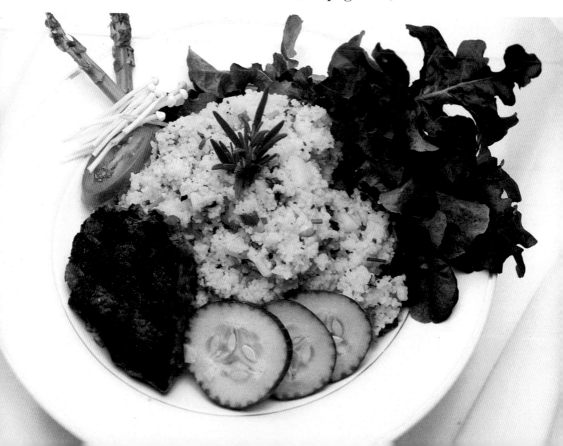

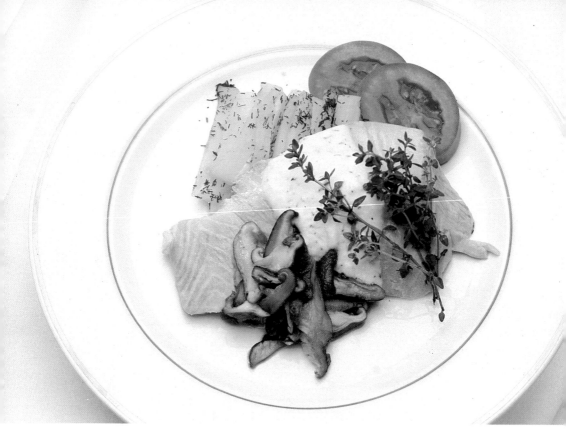

Poached Atlantic Salmon (see page 156)

Chicken Almond Stirfry (see page 153)

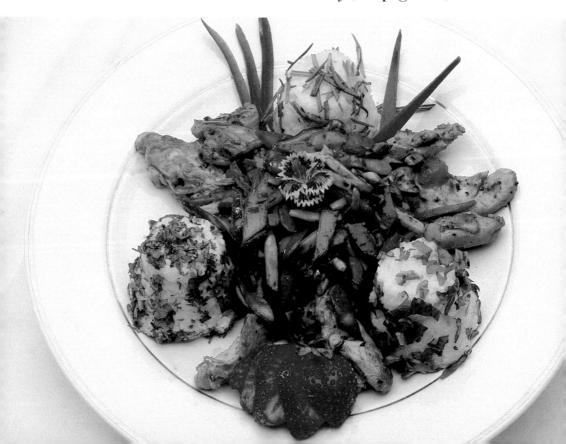

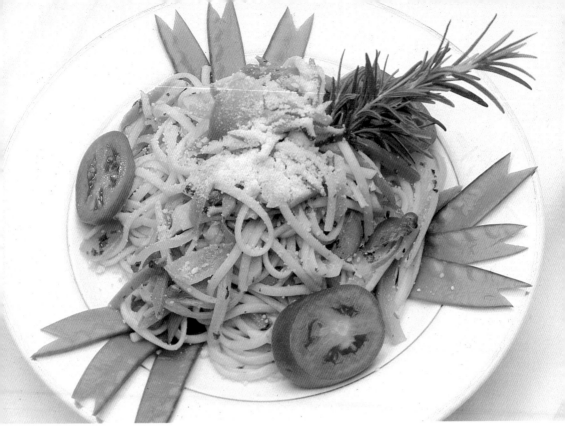

Linguini and Julienne Vegetables (see page 162)

Herb Baked Canadian Pickerel (see page 156)

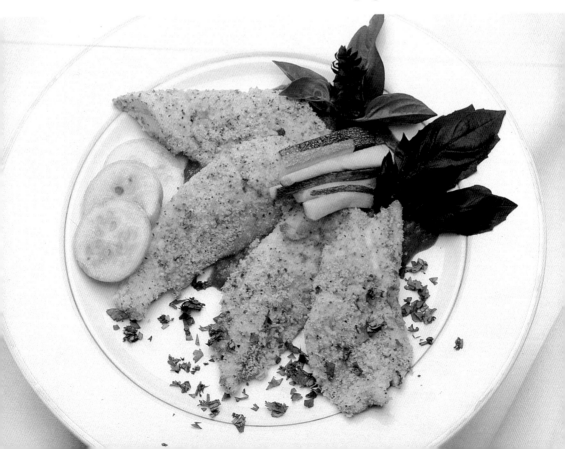

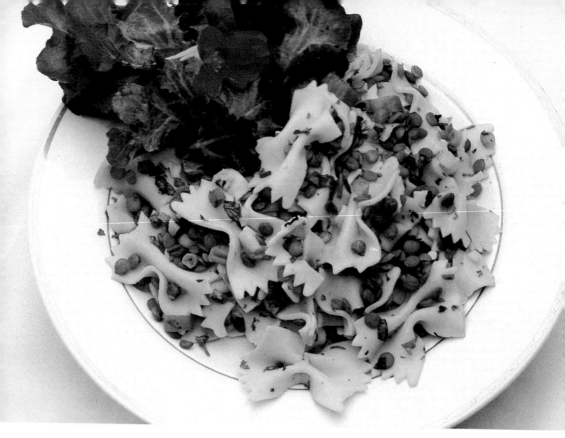

Farfella with Sweet Basil and Lentils (see page 162)

Pecan Breast of Chicken (see page 155)

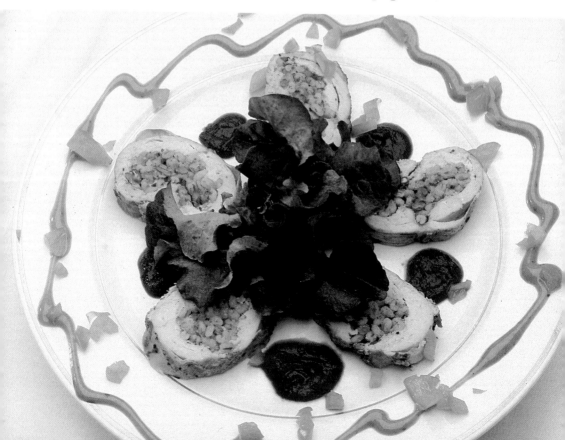

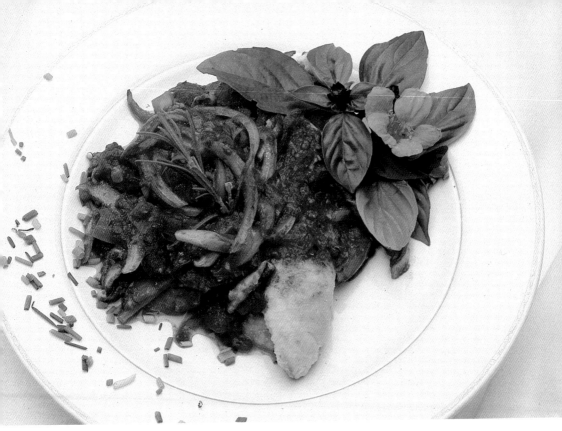

Creole Catfish (see page 157)

Charbroiled Halibut Steak (see page 157)

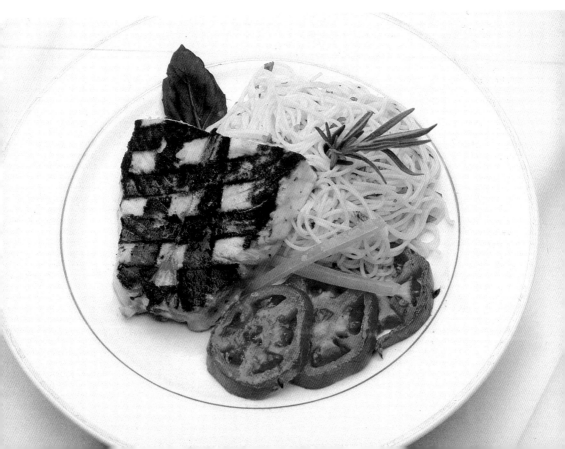

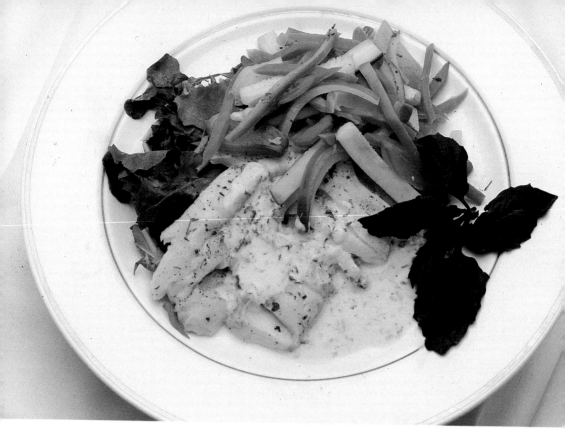

Oven Poached Scrod (see page 158)

Grilled Eggplant with Angel Hair Pasta (see page 161)

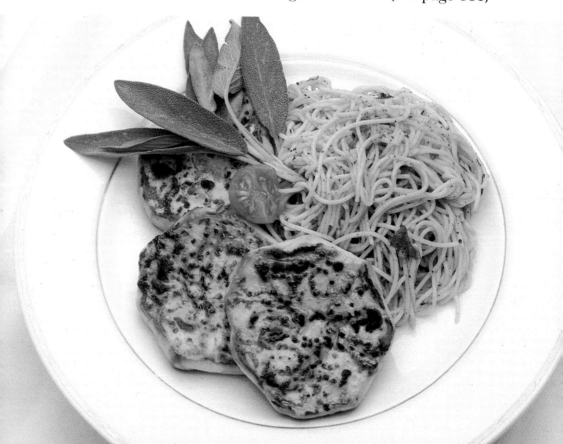

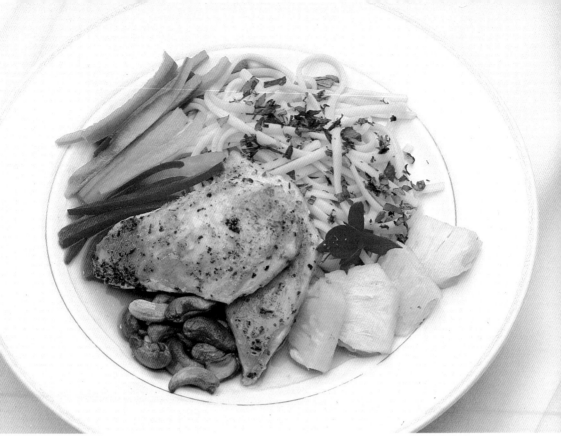

Gingered Cashew Chicken (see page 154)

Poached Stuffed Breast of Chicken (see page 154)

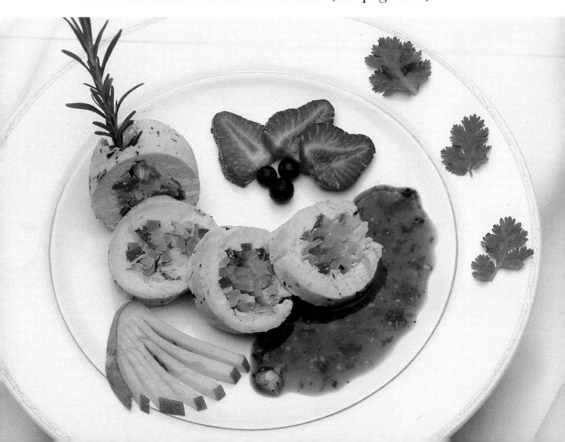

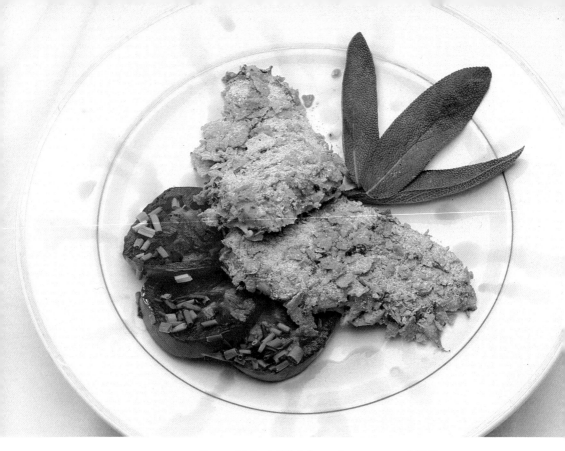

Oven Fried Chicken (see page 152)

Marinated Asparagus Spears (see page 146)

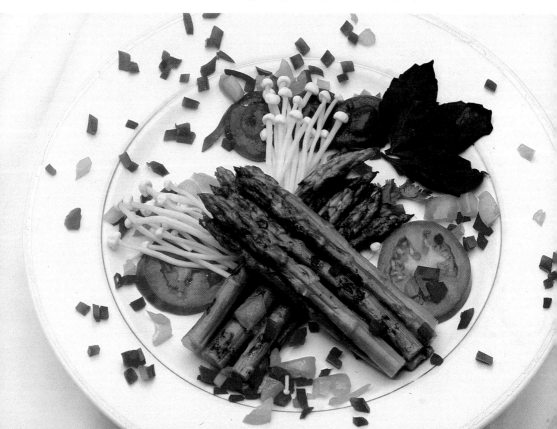

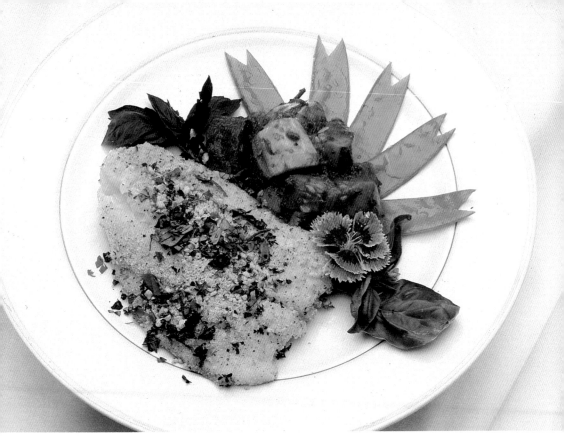

Cashew Crusted Orange Roughy (see page 158)

Grilled Sea Scallops (see page 159)

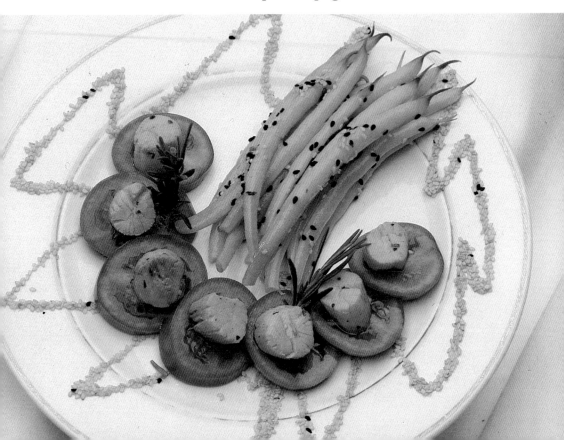

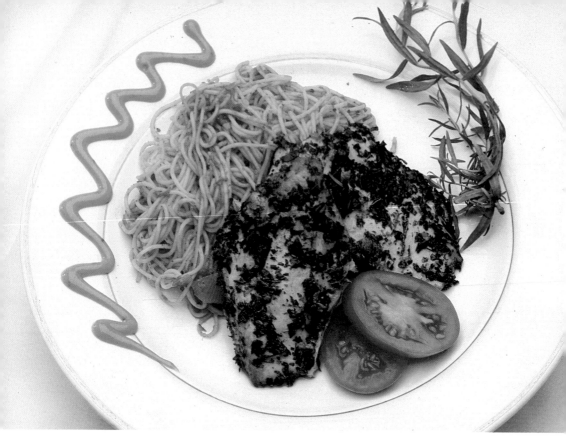

Chicken Breast Northcoast (see page 153)

Apple Cobbler (see page 170)

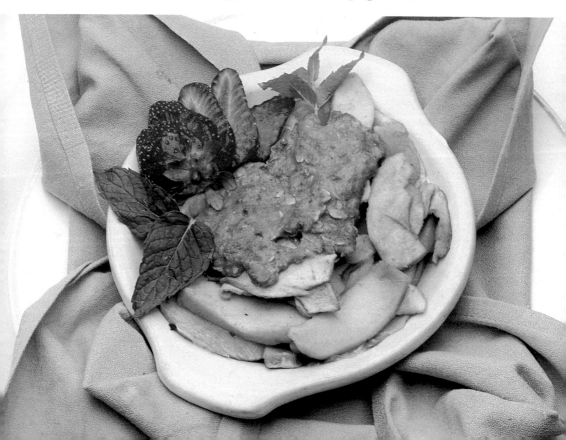

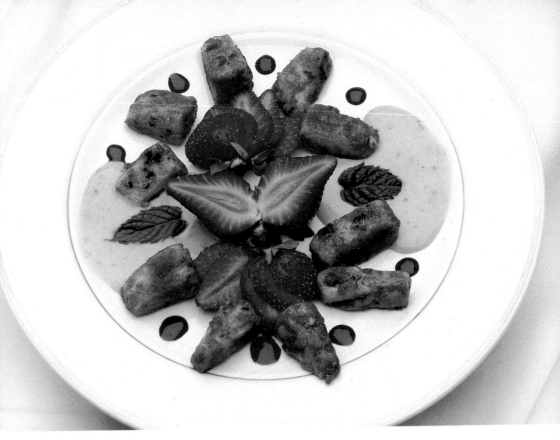

Sauteed Pineapple with Strawberry Yogurt Sauce (see page 168)

Poached Bartlett Pear (see page 168)

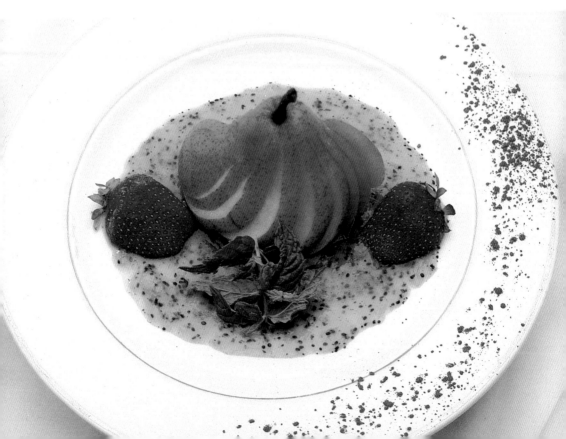

APPETIZER, SOUP AND SALAD RECIPES

Any good meal presentation begins with pre-dinner beverage and appetizers. Not only do they whet your appetite for the good food to follow, the cocktail hour is a simply delightful time of socializing. Friends talk of bygone days, business relationships build and grow, families get current on happenings with the clan and everyone has a grand time of laughs and refreshment. Good, tasty appetizers and drinks add so much to the pleasant atmosphere, and now they can be healthy as well.

So forget the fat-laden meatballs, sausages and dips. Here are low or no-fat recipes for a fun, enjoyable evening.

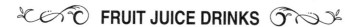 **FRUIT JUICE DRINKS**

BERRY-BANANA DELIGHT
Serves 1

½ Banana	1T Honey
8 Strawberries	1½ Scoops of Ice
½ Carton fat-free blueberry yogurt	

Mix in blender until smooth. Garnish with a strawberry with stem sliced, place on rim of glass.

STRAWBERRY-YOGURT SMOOTHIE
Serves 1

½ Banana
8 Strawberries

½ Carton fat-free strawberry yogurt
1½ Scoops of Ice

Mix in blender until smooth. Garnish with a banana slice and whole strawberry on a sword pick.

CASCADE COLADA
Serves 1

1 C Pineapple
½ Banana
½ C Cantaloupe

1 pkg. Sugar in the raw
½ C Apple juice
2 Scoops of Ice

Mix in blender until smooth. Garnish with a cantaloupe slice and whole strawberry on a sword pick.

HONEYDEW HONEY
Serves 1

1 C Honeydew
½ C Plain fat-free yogurt
½ Banana

½ Orange - squeezed
1 T Honey

Mix in blender until smooth. Garnish with a honeydew slice and strawberry on a sword pick.

APPLE FRAPPE
Serves 1

1 Apple - cored (save a slice
    for garnish)
1 C Apple juice
½ Orange - squeezed

½ Lemon - squeezed
1 pkg. sugar in the raw
1½ Scoops of Ice

Mix in blender until smooth. Garnish with an apple slice and strawberry on a sword pick.

APPETIZERS, SOUPS AND SALADS

QUICK FRUIT AND FIBER SNACK

8 oz. Assorted fruit:
    strawberries
    cantaloupe

1 T low-fat granola
½ C fat-free flavored yogurt

red and green grapes
watermelon
pineapple

Combine all fruit together and toss with the yogurt and low-fat granola. Serve.

CHICKEN SATAY APPETIZER
Serves 2

1 - 5 oz. boneless chicken breast
cut into 6 strips
1 tsp. low-sodium soy sauce
or Bragg's Aminos
1 tsp. chopped ginger

1 tsp. minced onion
½ tsp. Chinese 5 spice
½ defatted beef stock
1 T low-sodium peanut butter
1 tsp. honey

1. Marinate chicken strips in soy sauce, ginger, onions and Chinese 5 spice for
10-15 minutes.
2. Skewer chicken on bamboo sticks.
3. Broil for 4-5 minutes or until done.
4. Bring beef stock to a boil, add peanut butter and honey. Reduce to proper
consistency.
5. Drizzle over chicken and serve with herbed rice pilaf.

PEPPER STEAK BARLEY SOUP
Serves 4

6 cups defatted beef stock
1 C low-sodium tomato juice
1 small onion - diced
3 stalks celery - diced
8 oz. button mushrooms - quartered

½ C cooked pearled barley
¼ tsp. ground black pepper
2 T arrowroot
3 oz. diced cooked lean beef
1 tsp. kosher salt

1. Bring defatted beef stock to a boil and add onions, celery, pepper, mushrooms,
salt, tomato juice and diced beef. Reduce to a simmer and cook for 40 minutes.
2. Cook barley in a separate pan. Rinse and set aside.
3. Taste soup and adjust seasoning. Add barley.
4. Dissolve arrowroot in water and add slowly to the soup. Bring back to a boil and
remove from the heat. Serve.

CHILLED FRUIT SOUP
Serves 4

1 12 oz. can of pitted bing cherries
6 oz. strawberries
4 oz. cantaloupe
4 oz. blueberries
4 oz. honeydew

2 T granulated sugar
1 tsp. cinnamon
¼ C orange juice
1 T grenadine

1. Drain cherries and reserve the liquid.
2. Puree the cherries, strawberries, cantaloupe, honeydew and blueberries in a blender.

3. Add pureed fruit to cherry liquid and add sugar, grenadine, orange juice and cinnamon.
4. Stir well to dissolve the sugar. Chill until ready to use.
5. Serve with a dollop of any fruit flavored fat-free yogurt and fresh mint as a garnish.

NOTE: You can substitute any fruit depending upon the season or personal taste.

VEGETABLE CHILI
3 quarts

½ C diced onions	1 T chili powder
½ C diced celery	1 T ground cumin
½ C diced carrots	2 T chopped garlic
½ C diced peppers	1 T Caribbean jerk seasoning
½ C corn	2 C low-sodium dark kidney
2 C vegetable stock	beans - rinsed
2 22 oz. cans crushed tomatoes	½ tsp. cayenne pepper
½ C tomato puree	1 tsp. ground black pepper
2 C low-sodium tomato juice	1 T Canola oil

1. Saute in non-stick pan the onions, celery, garlic, carrots, and peppers in canola oil until tender.
2. Add crushed tomatoes, vegetable stock, tomato puree and tomato juice. Bring to a boil. Reduce to a simmer and cook for 45 minutes.
3. Add remaining ingredients and cook for 30 minutes. Adjust seasoning and serve over fat-free or vegetable hot dogs. Serve with additional onions, stadium or stone ground mustard. Also use any toppings that you and your family like. Add 1/2 lb of ground turkey and 1 lb noodles to make an entree.

HEARTY FIVE BEAN SOUP
Serves 8

½ C navy beans	4 celery stalks - diced
½ C turtle beans	2 carrots - diced
½ C pinto beans	3 quarts defatted chicken stock
½ C split peas	2 T marjoram
½ C lentils	2 tsp. kosher salt
1 medium onion - diced	½ tsp. black pepper

1. Soak navy, turtle and pinto beans overnight in water.
2. Drain soaked beans completely. Add chicken stock and bring to a boil. Reduce heat to a simmer. Add onions, celery and carrots. Cook for 45 minutes or until beans are 3/4 cooked.
3. Add lentils and split peas and cook for 30 more minutes or until tender.
4. Remove 1/2 of the bean mixture and puree in a blender. Add back to the original pot and add seasonings.
5. Serve with low-fat crackers or oven-baked corn chips.

QUICK ORIENTAL EGG DROP SOUP
Serves 2

1 can low-sodium, low-fat
   chicken vegetable soup
½ C chopped green onions

1 egg white
1 tsp sesame oil

1. Heat soup as can directs. Bring to a boil and add green onions. Reduce heat and simmer for 5 minutes.
2. When soup is done cooking, add egg white that has been gently whipped.
3. Remove from the heat and add sesame oil. Serve.

CASABLANCA TURKEY SALAD
Serves 2

8 oz. diced cooked turkey
   breast meat
2 T chopped green onions
2 T chopped celery
2 tsp. curry powder
¼ C low-fat cottage cheese
¼ C non-fat mayonnaise

1 T tarragon vinegar
1 T low-fat plain yogurt
1 T chopped parsley
1 T brandy
3 oz. field greens
1 medium tomato, cut in wedges
salt to taste if desired

1. Combine turkey, green onions, celery and curry powder. Mix well.
2. In a blender, whip cottage cheese until smooth and add mayonnaise, vinegar, yogurt, parsley and brandy.
3. Mix dressing with the turkey mixture and toss gently.
4. Place on a chilled plate with tomato wedges and field greens.

OPTIONAL: Can drizzle any flavored fat-free dressing you like over the field greens.

CHICKEN WALDORF SALAD
Serves 1

3 C red delicious apples -
   peeled, cored and diced
3 T non-fat mayonnaise
2 T plain fat-free yogurt
¼ C diced celery
1 T raisins

1 T dried cherries
1 T chopped walnuts
½ C diced cooked chicken breast
3 strawberries
1 sprig fresh mint garnish

1. In a bowl, combine yogurt, mayonnaise, raisins, cherries, celery and walnuts.
2. Mix chicken and apples together.
3. Pour dressing over apple chicken mixture and gently toss.
4. Serve with fluted strawberries and fresh mint.

CHICKEN AND ARTICHOKE SALAD
Serves 4

8 oz. cooked julienne chicken breast   1 T chopped parsley

1 14 oz. can whole artichokes -
   drained and chopped
1 T minced shallots
2 T chopped green onions
2 T diced roasted red peppers
   or pimientos

½ C non-fat mayonnaise
1 T plain low-fat yogurt
1 T fat-free ranch dressing
1 T chopped fresh tarragon
1 T tarragon vinegar
16 pieces of romaine hearts

1. Combine julienne chicken breast, artichokes, shallots, green onions and roasted red peppers.
2. In a bowl, whisk together non-fat mayonnaise, parsley, plain low-fat yogurt, fat-free ranch dressing, fresh tarragon and tarragon vinegar.
3. Pour dressing over the chicken mixture and toss gently.
4. Place romaine leaves towards the top of the plate and line the bottom with the chicken mixture.
5. Garnish with fresh thyme and paprika.

GERMAN TOMATO AND CUCUMBER SALAD
Serves 2

4 large tomatoes, diced and drained
2 T chopped chives or scallions
½ C low-sodium smoked turkey
1 scored English cucumber - sliced
2 T chopped dill
sprig of fresh dill

¼ C non-fat mayonnaise
¼ C fat-free plain yogurt
¼ C imitation sour cream
juice of 1 lime
salt to taste if desired
¼ tsp. white pepper

1. Mix together tomatoes, chives and smoked turkey.
2. In a small bowl combine mayonnaise, yogurt, sour cream and lime juice.
3. Pour over tomato mix and toss gently.
4. Arrange sliced cucumbers on plate in a circle and place tomato mix in the middle.
5. Serve with appropriate garnish.

SPICY NAPA COLE SLAW

2 heads of napa cabbage -
   thinly sliced
1 carrot - shredded
5 scallions - sliced
½ C non-fat mayonnaise
1 T sugar

½ C non-fat plain yogurt
¼ C tarragon vinegar
1 T Caribbean jerk seasoning
1 T black sesame seeds
1 tsp. cayenne pepper

1. Combine cabbage, carrots and scallions. Mix well.
2. In a separate bowl, combine mayonnaise, yogurt, tarragon vinegar, sesame seeds, cayenne pepper, sugar and jerk seasoning.
3. Pour over cabbage mixture and combine well. Chill prior to serving.

CHARBROILED ROMA TOMATO SALAD
Serves 2

6 ½ inch slices of tomato
2 T fat free Italian dressing
1 tsp. saltless table seasoning
1 T julienne red pepper
1 T julienne yellow pepper

1 T julienne green pepper
2 radicchio leaves
2 sprigs of fresh tarragon
2 bunches of enoki mushrooms

1. Marinate tomato slices with dressing for 2 minutes.
2. Grill 1 minute on each side.
3. Place on plate with radicchio.
4. Sprinkle diced peppers on top and garnish with fresh tarragon and enoki mushrooms.

SHRIMP AND BARLEY SALAD
Serves 2

6 medium pieces cooked
    frozen shrimp
4 C cooked barley
½ C diced roasted red peppers
½ C green onions - cut on a bias
½ C diced cantaloupe
2 T chopped cilantro
½ C nonfat lemon dill dressing

juice of 2 limes
2 T ground cumin
½ T black pepper
1 tsp. kosher salt
3 T chopped parsley
¾ C apple cider vinegar
1 cucumber, medium - sliced

1. Mix all ingredients together except shrimp.
2. Line a plate with sliced cucumbers and place barley mixture in the middle of the plate.
3. Garnish around with the pieces of shrimp.

BANANA PEPPERS AND SPINACH SALAD
Serves 4

8 banana peppers - stems and
    seeds removed
1 C julienne red onions
1 T olive oil
1 T chopped garlic
1 C red wine vinegar

½ T crushed red peppers
1 T chopped basil
1 tsp. kosher salt
½ tsp. ground black pepper
1 lb. leaf spinach

1. Heat oil in pan until very hot, add peppers and onions. Cook 5-7 minutes.
2. Add salt, black pepper, red pepper and basil. Cook 1 minute.
3. Add red wine vinegar, stir in and remove from heat. Cover and let sit for 1 hour.
4. When chilled, mix with leaf spinach and serve as a salad course.

PLEASE TELL YOUR GUESTS THAT THE PEPPERS ARE VERY HOT.

GRILLED SHRIMP AND WARM VEGETABLE SALAD CAPELLINI

4 lunch portions

Two pounds of the following vegetables (can substitute any vegetables that you like):

white mushrooms
carrots
bell peppers
yellow squash
onion pieces
broccoli florets
cauliflower
zucchini

1 lb. capellini (angel hair)
1 lb. peeled and deveined shrimp
1 C fat-free lemon herb dressing
2 T basil
2 T oregano

1. Cut all vegetables into 1-2 inch pieces. Poach or steam until cooked tender. Cool and drain.
2. Marinate chilled vegetables in fat-free lemon herb dressing. Add fresh basil and oregano to the marinade. Amounts depend on your own personal taste. Marinate overnight.
3. Cook pasta until done, rinse in hot water and drain. Place equal amounts on 4 plates and reserve.
4. Cook vegetables on broiler until warm, turning one time to keep from burning. Add some remaining vegetable marinade to the shrimp and place on the griddle or a non-stick pan.
5. Remove vegetables from the broiler and place on top of the pasta. Add shrimp when done.
6. Serve with a side of fat-free dressing.

15

ENTREE AND VEGETABLE RECIPES

Sumptuous chicken, grilled fish, charbroiled steaks and mounds of succulent vegetables make up the bulk of the Biotech Eating Plan. Other weight management methods shy away from such great eating, but not us.

Chef Edward has designed recipes that look good, taste great and fill up your dinner plate. No tiny and delicate "Nouvelle Cuisine" portions here. This is American food, and plenty of it, made just for American appetites. Best of all, it's low-fat, high in complex carbohydrates and good for you. So go ahead — indulge yourself.

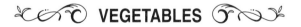 **VEGETABLES**

RED BEANS AND RICE
Serves 6-8 people

2 cans red beans - soaked	2 C cooked rice
6 C defatted chicken stock	1 T chopped garlic
2 T chopped onion	1 tsp. black pepper
2 T chopped celery	1 tsp. cayenne pepper
2 T chopped peppers	1 T canola oil
½ T chopped jalepenos	1 tsp. kosher salt

1. Saute garlic, onions, celery and peppers until tender.

2. Add drained red beans and chicken stock. Cook until 3/4 done. Add the jalepenos and finish cooking.
3. Add cooked rice, black pepper, salt and cayenne pepper. Cook for 2 minutes and serve.

CAN BE MADE MANY DAYS AHEAD AND REHEATED IN THE MICROWAVE OVEN WITHOUT ADDING ANY FAT.

HERBED RICE PILAF
Serves 6

2 T chopped onion	2 C defatted chicken stock
2 T chopped bell peppers	1 T chopped parsley
2 T chopped mushrooms	1 T chopped basil
1 T chopped garlic	1 T chopped thyme
1 tsp. canola oil	1 tsp. kosher salt
1 C converted rice - rinsed	

1. Saute onions in canola oil with peppers, mushrooms and garlic until transparent.
2. Add rinsed rice and saute for 2-3 minutes.
3. Add chicken stock, parsley, basil, thyme and salt. Bring to a boil while stirring. Reduce to a simmer, cover and cook 15 minutes.
4. Remove from the heat and serve.

MARINATED NORTHERN AND TURTLE BEANS
Serves 10-12

3 C cooked northern beans	2 T minced shallots
3 C turtle or black beans	2 T chopped parsley
1 C fat free italian salad dressing	1 T saltless table seasoning

1. Combine all ingredients, mix well and chill until ready to serve.

BAKED ACORN SQUASH
Serves 4

1 large acorn squash	1 tsp. pumpkin pie spice
¼ C brown sugar	1 T lemon juice
¼ C honey	

1. Cut squash in half and scoop all of the seeds out. Cut in quarters.
2. Place flesh side down in a baking pan with 2 cups of water. Bake in 350° oven for 1 hour.
3. Remove from the oven and turn squash over. Baste with brown sugar, honey lemon juice and pumpkin pie spice 3 - 4 times while still baking. Soak for 10-15 minutes more.
4. Remove from oven and serve.

ACORN SQUASH CAN BE COOKED THE DAY BEFORE AND CHILLED. THIS PREPARATION CAN BE DONE VERY QUICKLY.

Oven Steamed Red Bliss Potatoes
Serves 4

12 red bliss potatoes	1 tsp. fresh ground black pepper
2 C defatted chicken stock	½ T fresh marjoram
2 T chopped chives	½ tsp. kosher salt

1. Place potatoes in a casserole dish and cover with chicken stock.
2. Add remaining ingredients on top.
3. Cover with lid or foil and bake in a 300° oven for 30 minutes or until done.

OPTIONAL: Butter flavored sprinkles can be added but remember they are high in sodium.

Oven Jerked French Fries
Serves 4

1 lb. washed and dried potatoes	1 tsp. jerk seasoning
¼ C egg whites	vegetable spray

1. Slice potato into julienne strips, leaving the skin on.
2. Coat with egg whites and season with jerk seasoning.
3. Bake on a cookie sheet sprayed with vegetable spray at 400° for 20 minutes. Turn often. Note: Oven temperatures vary so you may need to modify cooking time.

Polenta, Mushrooms and Marinara Sauce
Serves 6

2 cups polenta	1 tsp. chopped garlic
4 cups defatted chicken stock	1 tsp. olive oil
1 cup sliced mushrooms	3 C marinara sauce
1 T minced shallots	3 oz. parmesan cheese

1. In a sauce pan, saute garlic, mushrooms and shallots in oil.
2. Add chicken stock and stir in polenta slowly, whipping all the time. This will eliminate lumping.
3. Bring polenta to a boil and cook for 8-10 minutes.
4. Heat marinara sauce in a separate pot.
5. Remove polenta from the heat and spread on top of a cutting board large enough to spread about 1/4 inch thick.
6. Spread marinara sauce on top and cover with cheese. Eat immediately.

Rattatouillie
Serves 8-10

2 onions, diced	1 T chopped garlic
2 bell peppers, diced	4 C low-sodium tomato juice
3 medium zucchini, diced	1 T chopped sweet basil
3 medium yellow squash, diced	1 T chopped parsley
4 tomatoes, diced	1 T chopped oregano

1 eggplant   1 T chopped thyme
1 T olive oil

1. Peel eggplant. Dice and cover completely in cool water to keep from turning brown.
2. Saute garlic in olive oil until golden brown. Do not overcook as it will turn bitter.
3. Add onions and cook for 5 minutes. Then add peppers and cook for 5 minutes.
4. Add zucchini and squash and cook for 5 more minutes. Add tomatoes, tomato juice and eggplant. Simmer for 30 minutes.
5. With 10 minutes left to cook, add the parsley, basil, thyme and oregano. Remove from the fire and cool quickly to retain as much color as possible.

MARINATED ASPARAGUS SPEARS
Serves 2

30 asparagus spears - fresh, steamed and chilled
6 mushroom caps, steamed and chilled

1 T diced red pepper
1 T diced yellow pepper
4 tomato slices
2 T fat-free herb dressing

1. Marinate asparagus and mushrooms for 5 minutes in fat-free herb dressing.
2. Charbroil briefly to get the charcoal flavor. Remove from grill.
3. Place tomato on a plate with 2 piles of asparagus (pile on like logs).
4. Arrange mushrooms and garnish with diced peppers.
5. Drizzle with extra dressing.

TWICE BAKED POTATO
Serves 4

4 baked potatoes
1 T chopped garlic
1 T minced shallots
¼ C skim milk
¼ C fat-free sour cream

½ C diced green onions
½ tsp. ground white pepper
¼ C vegetable stock
1 T chopped parsley

1. Combine garlic and shallots with the vegetable stock and poach until tender. Drain.
2. Scoop out the insides of the potato and place in a bowl. Mash very well before adding anything else. This will help to get out any lumps.
3. Add garlic, shallots, skim milk, sour cream, green onions, white pepper and parsley. Mix completely.
4. Add mix back into the hollowed out potato and bake in the oven at 350° for 5-7 minutes.

BRAISED FENNEL
Serves 6

6 C sliced fresh fennel bulb
1 C julienne onions
2 C basic vegetable stock

½ T canola oil
2 T chopped fresh fennel sprigs
1 T chopped fresh parsley

1. Saute the onions in canola oil until transparent. Add sliced fennel and saute 3-5 minutes.
2. Add vegetable stock, bring to a boil, reduce heat to a slow simmer and cover with a lid. Cook for about 15 minutes or until tender.
3. When fennel is tender, add chopped fennel sprigs and parsley. Serve hot or at room temperature.

VEGETABLE KABOBS
Serves 4

4 12 inch bamboo skewers	4 green peppers, 1 x 1 square
8 zucchini pieces, 1½ x 1½	4 red pearl onions
8 squash pieces, 1½ x 1½	4 white pearl onions
4 cherry tomatoes	½ C fat free Italian dressing
4 whole button mushrooms	¼ C white wine
4 yellow peppers, 1 x 1 square	½ T saltless seasoning
4 red peppers, 1 x 1 square	

1. Skewer evenly all the ingredients. Make sure you alternate the colors to make an attractive presentation.
2. Marinate in dressing for 10 minutes and charbroil until done.

Vegetables may be poached prior to skewering to make it easier. Use your imagination and add shrimp, scallops or chicken and follow the same idea. Change this from a vegetable to a fabulous dinner presentation.

JULIENNE VEGETABLE CHOW MEIN
Serves 4

1 C julienne snow peas	1 T olive oil
1 C julienne carrots	1 T minced shallots
½ C julienne leeks	1 T chopped garlic
½ C julienne red peppers	1 T chopped ginger
½ C julienne waterchestnuts	1½ tsp. sesame oil
½ C julienne shiitake	2 T plum sauce
mushrooms	2 T low-sodium soy sauce
½ C julienne bok choy	¼ C defatted chicken stock
(chinese cabbage)	3 tsp. cornstarch
½ C green onions -	2 T saki (Japanese rice wine)
diagonal cut	1 lb. cooked lo mein noodles or linguini

1. Place oil in a wok and heat. When hot, saute very quickly the shallots, garlic and ginger for 1-2 minutes.
2. Add snow peas, carrots, leeks, red peppers, waterchestnuts, shiitake mushrooms and bok choy. Cook until tender.
3. Add sesame oil, plum sauce, chicken stock, soy sauce and lo mein noodles. Toss gently.
4. Dissolve cornstarch in saki and add just before removing from the heat. Cook for 1 minute.

SPINACH AND BEAN ENCHILADAS
Serves 4

2-16 oz. cans cooked low-sodium
pinto beans - rinsed and drained
¼ C minced onions
½ T chopped garlic
1 T chili powder
½ T cumin

8 flour tortillas
4 T fat-free sour cream
1 C green chili salsa
½ C low-fat shredded jack cheese
spinach leaves

1. Drain and rinse pinto beans. Mash until smooth.
2. Add garlic, onions, chili powder and cumin.
3. Line tortilla shell with spinach leaves and place pinto beans inside. Roll up and place in a baking pan.
4. Cover with green chili salsa and bake in a 350° oven for 10 minutes or until hot.
5. Remove from the oven and top with cheese. Place back in the oven until cheese melts.
6. Garnish with fat-free sour cream.

EGGPLANT PARMESAN
Serves 6

6 eggplant slices, 1 - 1½ inches thick
1 C basic marinara sauce
6 oz. white bread crumbs
1 tsp. paprika

1 tsp. chopped basil
1 tsp. chopped oregano
1 tsp. chopped thyme
2 T kosher salt

1. Peel and slice 1 medium eggplant into 6 slices. Coat with salt and refrigerate overnight. This will remove the bitter flavor of the eggplant.
2. Rinse the eggplant very well and pat dry.
3. In a bowl combine bread crumbs, paprika, basil, oregano, thyme and parmesan cheese.
4. Grill the eggplant in a non-stick pan very quickly. Remove to a baking dish.
5. Ladle sauce over the eggplant and top with bread crumb mixture. Bake in a 350° oven for 15-20 minutes or until golden brown and tender.

THE DELMONTE
Serves 2

3 lbs. green and white
asparagus stems
12 button or shiitake mushrooms
¼ C diced red peppers

¼ C diced green pepper
¼ C diced yellow peppers
1 tomato - sliced
½ C fat-free dressing - Italian or similar

1. Steam fresh asparagus until tender. Place in ice water to stop cooking and retain color.
2. Steam the mushrooms just like in step 1.
3. Marinate asparagus and mushrooms in dressing for 10-15 minutes.
4. Place tomato slices on plate with the asparagus. Line up mushrooms and sprinkle diced peppers as garnish.
5. Drizzle extra dressing on the plate and serve.
6. Serve well-chilled.

SPICY SPANISH OMELETTE
Serves 1

1 T diced onion
1 T diced bell peppers
1 T diced tomatoes
1 T chives
1 T cooked potatoes (can use leftover baked potatoes)

2 T low-sodium tomato juice
1 tsp. minced garlic
¼ tsp. cayenne pepper
2 shakes Tabasco
¾ C fat-free egg substitute
vegetable spray

1. Saute onions, tomatoes, tomato juice, peppers, garlic and potatoes in a non-stick pan.
2. Add cayenne pepper and Tabasco to the eggs and pour into the saute pan with the vegetable mixture.
3. As the eggs begin to cook, shake the pan and rotate the cooked egg to the center of the pan allowing the uncooked egg mix to move to the outside of the pan.
4. When the majority of the eggs are cooked, flip over with a spatula. Cook a little more and then roll out onto a plate.

GRILLED VEGETARIAN SANDWICH WITH WHOLE WHEAT PITA BREAD
Serves 1

1 oz julienne onion
1 oz julienne bell peppers
1 oz julienne celery
1 oz sliced mushrooms
1 oz bean sprouts
1 oz diced tofu

1 oz alfalfa sprouts
1 oz julienne snow peas
1 oz diced tomatoes
3 oz shredded lettuce
2 T fat-free Italian dressing
1 whole wheat pita

1. Combine onions, peppers, celery, mushrooms, bean sprouts, tofu, and snow peas with salad dressing.
2. Grill on a non-stick griddle or pan until tender (2-3 minutes).
3. Slice the tip off the pita bread and put into the toaster.
4. Add lettuce to the bottom of the pita and place cooked mixture over the lettuce. Top with alfalfa sprouts and diced tomatoes.
5. Serve with spicy napa cabbage and boiled red bliss potatoes with chives.

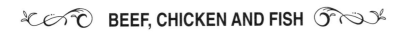 **BEEF, CHICKEN AND FISH**

GRILLED TENDERLOIN OF BEEF AND COUSCOUS
Serves 2

2 - 2½ oz. tenderloin medallions
4 C cooked couscous
1 C diced tomatoes
1 C diced cucumbers, seedless and skinless
½ C fat-free tangerine mint dressing

¼ C fresh chopped mint
¼ C chopped parsley
2 T lemon juice
½ T minced garlic
1 tsp. ground cumin
salt and pepper to taste

1. Prepare couscous as directed on the package. Just remember to use defatted

chicken stock to cook with.

2. In a bowl, combine couscous, tomatoes, cucumbers, orange mint dressing, parsley, lemon juice, garlic, cumin, salt and pepper.

3. Charbroil medallion to desired temperature and serve with couscous and garnish as desired.

SAUTEED BEEF MEDALLIONS AND JICAMA

Serves 2

2-2 ½ oz. beef medallions
4 oz. sliced mushrooms
1 T chopped garlic
1 T chopped shallots
1 T dijon mustard
6 oz. defatted beef stock

1 T arrowroot
6 oz. jicama - julienne
1 tsp. saltless table seasoning
4 oz. red wine
5 oz. rotini pasta

1. Saute beef medallions in non-stick pan sprayed with vegetable spray.
2. When half way done add garlic, mushrooms and shallots.
3. Add red wine and reduce by 1/2. Add beef stock and continue cooking.
4. Stir in mustard and rotini, thicken with arrowroot.
5. Grill jicama separately and garnish medallions. Serve.

REDUCED FAT HAMBURGER

Serves 6

1 lb. ground beef, extra lean
1 C textured vegetable
   protein (T.V.P.)
½ C water
2 T tomato paste
2 T chopped parsley
2 tsp. saltless seasoning

6 tomato slices
6 lettuce leaves
6 whole wheat,
   split hamburger buns
fat-free mayo - optional
low-fat cheese - optional

1. Soak vegetable protein in water and set aside for 10 minutes.
2. Combine paste, parsley, seasoning and ground beef with the vegetable protein. Form 6 patties and grill as usual. Serve with oven jerked french fries.
3. If you wish to reduce the fat content even more, you can add additional protein as you wish. NOTE: T.V.P. can be purchased in bulk from any good health food store.

COUSCOUS AND GRILLED ONION HAMBURGER

Serves 6

1 lb. ground beef, extra lean
8 oz. cooked couscous
1 tsp. chopped garlic
1 tsp. chopped shallots
¼ C tomato juice
1 T chopped parsley
1 T Heinz 57 sauce

6 slices of tomato
6 leaves of lettuce
low-fat cheese - optional
fat-free mayonnaise - optional
1 medium onion - julienne
6 whole wheat hamburger buns, split

1 Cook couscous and set aside to chill completely.
2. Combine the ground beef, garlic, shallots, tomato juice, parsley, Heinz 57 sauce and chilled couscous.
3. Form 6 patties and grill as usual.
4. When hamburgers are cooking, grill onions until golden brown and serve on top of each burger.
5. Serve with oven jerked french fries.

STADIUM PEARLBURGER
Serves 6

1 lb. ground beef - extra lean	6 lettuce leaves
8 oz. cooked pearled barley	2 C sliced mushrooms
2 egg whites	low-fat cheese - optional
3 T A-1 steak sauce	fat-free mayonnaise - optional
2 T stadium mustard	6 whole wheat split hamburger buns
6 slices tomato	

1. Cook barley separately, drain and set aside to cool.
2. Combine the ground hamburger, steak sauce, stadium mustard, egg whites and barley.
3. Form into patties and grill as desired.
4. When hamburgers are cooking, grill the mushrooms and serve on top of the burgers.
5. Serve with oven jerked french fries.

GROUND TURKEY BURGER
Serves 4

1 lb. ground turkey breast	2 oz. of part-skim, low-fat
2 egg whites	mozzarella cheese
2 T minced shallots	8 slices cracked whole wheat,
2 T chopped parsley	low-sodium bread
4 oz. cranberry apple relish	1 lb. assorted fresh fruit

1. Combine ground turkey, egg whites, shallots and parsley. Mix together well.
2. Cook in a hot, non-stick pan until almost done. Add mozzarella cheese and melt.
3. Serve on cracked whole wheat bread with cranberry apple relish and assorted fresh fruit.

TURKEY MEAT LOAF
Serves 6

1 lb. ground turkey breast, no skin	1 C cooked pearled barley
½ C shredded zucchini	¼ C egg whites
½ C shredded carrots	2 T stone ground mustard
½ C yellow squash	1 tsp. saltless seasoning
½ C diced green onions	2 tsp. Heinz 57 Sauce
1 T chopped garlic	½ C defatted chicken stock

1. Saute the garlic and onions in a non-stick pan with vegetable spray until tender. Add zucchini, squash and carrots. Cook until tender, about 2-3 minutes. Set aside and let cool.
2. Combine in a bowl the turkey, barley, egg whites, mustard, Heinz 57 and chicken stock.
3. Add cooked mixture and mix completely.
4. Place in a loaf pan and bake at 350° until internal temperature reaches 170°. Do not overcook as this product will dry out.
5. Remove from the oven and let cool for 5 minutes before slicing. Serve with your choice of side dishes.
6. Serve with marinara sauce or parmesan dill dip.

TURKEY PARMESAN WITH OVEN ROASTED MARINARA SAUCE
Serves 4

8 - 2 oz. thinly sliced raw turkey breasts	1 tsp. saltless table seasoning
¼ C all purpose flour	1¼ C roasted vegetable marinara sauce (see recipe)
2 T egg whites	2 oz. part-skim low-fat mozzarella cheese, paprika to season.
1 C sifted dried bread crumbs	
2 oz. parmesan cheese	

1. Season turkey breasts with saltless seasoning. Dredge in flour and place in the egg whites.
2. Combine bread crumbs and parmesan cheese. Add turkey to the bread mix and coat completely.
3. Place on a baking sheet with silicone paper and bake in a 350° oven for 5-7 minutes or until done.
4. Remove from the oven. Ladle marinara sauce over and cover with mozzarella cheese. Sprinkle with paprika and place back in the oven for just a few minutes to melt and brown the cheese.

OVEN FRIED CHICKEN BREAST
Serves 2

2 - 6 oz. boneless chicken breasts	¼ tsp. onion powder
¼ C crushed corn flakes	1 T fresh chives - diced
1 T flour	1 egg white - whipped
¼ tsp. garlic powder	8 tomato slices
¼ tsp. cayenne pepper	¼ T hot chili oil
¼ tsp. dried parsley	

1. Combine corn flakes, flour, garlic powder, onion powder, cayenne pepper and parsley.
2. Cut chicken breasts in half and place on a baking sheet covered with silicone paper.
3. Brush chicken breast with whipped egg white and coat with the corn flake mixture.
4. Bake in a 375° oven for 15 minutes or until done.
5. Remove from the oven and place on top of sliced grilled tomatoes. Drizzle with hot chili oil and garnish with fresh chives.

STUFFED CHICKEN BREAST NORTHCOAST WITH TOMATO BASIL SAUCE
Serves 2

2 - 6 oz. boneless chicken breasts	1 tsp. saltless seasoning
4 oz. julienne carrots	1 onion - sliced
6 spinach leaves	5 oz. tomato basil sauce
½ T minced shallots	

1. Poach carrots halfway done. Poach spinach for 30 seconds.
2. Saute shallots for 1 minute in a non-stick pan.
3. Pound out chicken breasts 1/2 larger than their original size. Rub with the cooked shallots.
4. Lay poached spinach on the chicken breast and lace julienne carrots lengthwise. Roll up tightly and place on a baking sheet with silicone paper.
5. Bake at 300° for 20 - 25 minutes or until done.
6. Grill onions on a non-stick surface until golden brown.
7. Remove chicken and let set for 5 minutes. Slice and plate up with tomato basil sauce and grilled onions.
8. Garnish as you desire.

CAN BE MADE THE DAY BEFORE WITHOUT LOSING FLAVOR. ALSO CAN BE FROZEN VERY NICELY FOR USE AT A LATER DATE.

CHARBROILED BONELESS BREAST OF CHICKEN WITH PINEAPPLE CHUTNEY
Serves 2

2 - 6 oz. boneless breasts	½ T canola oil
½ T saltless table seasoning	5 oz. pineapple chutney

1. Season chicken and rub in oil.
2. Charbroil chicken until done. Remove from fire and cut in half.
3. Serve with pineapple chutney and fruit garnish.

CHICKEN ALMOND STIR FRY
Serves 2

1 - 6 oz. boneless chicken breast, cut into strips	½ T chopped garlic
2 oz. julienne red onion	½ T minced shallots
2 oz. julienne carrots	2 tsp. low sodium soy sauce
2 oz. julienne snow peas	1 T sesame oil
2 oz. julienne mushrooms	2 T plum sauce
2 oz. julienne waterchestnuts	2 T slivered almonds
2 oz. bean sprouts	1 tsp. soybean oil
1 T fresh ginger	2 tsp. Chinese 5 spice

1. Heat wok and add soybean oil. Work quickly at this time!!!
2. Add garlic and shallots. Cook for 1-2 minutes. Leave on low heat.
3. Add chicken and cook until 3/4 of the way done. Add onions, carrots, snow peas, mushrooms and water chestnuts.
4. Cook until chicken is done.
5. Add remaining ingredients and serve with herbed rice.

GINGERED CASHEW CHICKEN
Serves 1

1 - 5 oz. boneless chicken breast
1½ oz. pineapple
1½ oz. julienne peppers
½ T chopped parsley
3 oz. demi-glaze
1 T cashews
½ tsp. sesame oil

½ tsp. low-sodium soy sauce
  or Bragg's Aminos
1 T diced fresh ginger
1 tsp. Chinese 5 Spice
1 T red currant jelly
2 oz. cooked lo mein noodles

1. Marinate boneless chicken breast in fresh ginger, sesame oil and soy sauce for 30 minutes.
2. Saute chicken breast in a non-stick pan on both sides until 3/4 done, about 6-8 minutes.
3. Add peppers and pineapple. Cook for 2 minutes.
4. Add demi-glaze, Chinese 5 spice, cashews and red currant jelly. Cook until desired consistency and the chicken is done.
5. Remove from the stove and serve with lo mein noodles and garnish.

POACHED STUFFED BONELESS BREAST OF CHICKEN
Serves 1

1 - 5 oz. boneless chicken breast
2 oz. julienne carrots, leeks,
  peppers, zucchini and squash
3 oz. wild field greens

2 oz. champagne balsamic vinaigrette
3 oz. defatted chicken stock
strawberries, blueberries and
  orange sections for garnish

1. Poach julienne vegetables in defatted chicken stock. Remove from liquid and let cool.
2. Pound out chicken breast to about 1/2 larger in size. Place julienne vegetables in the middle and roll up tightly.
3. Wrap chicken in plastic wrap to keep its shape. Poach about 15 minutes in the same liquid that the vegetables were cooked in.
4. Remove chicken and let cool briefly.
5. Place wild greens on a plate and slice chicken into 6-8 slices and place on top of the greens.
6. Garnish with strawberries, blueberries and orange sections.
7. Drizzle with champagne balsamic vinaigrette and serve.

GRILLED BREAST OF CHICKEN PALOMBO
Serves 2

2 - 5 oz boneless chicken breast
1 T fresh chopped basil
1 T fresh chopped oregano
1 T fresh chopped parsley
½ T fresh chopped garlic

2 C of cooked angel hair pasta
1 C marinara sauce
1 tsp. saltless table seasoning
1 tsp. olive oil
6 oz. zucchini

1. Rub and coat chicken breasts completely with basil, oregano, garlic and parsley.
2. Heat non-stick pan with olive oil. Get very hot and sear both sides of the chicken. Place in the oven for 10-12 minutes or until done.

3. Remove from oven and let cool for 5 minutes.
4. Slice and serve with angel hair marinara.
5. Use zucchini as a garnish - slice and grill on a bias.

BARLEY AND PECAN BREAST OF CHICKEN
Serves 2

2 - 5 oz. boneless chicken breasts	1 T honey
5 oz. cooked barley	2 T egg whites
3 oz. pecans	½ tsp. cinnamon
1 T brown sugar	½ tsp. nutmeg

1. Pound out chicken breasts until 1/2 larger in size.
2. Combine barley, pecans, brown sugar, honey, cinnamon, egg whites and nutmeg.
3. Place in the middle of the chicken breast and roll up tightly.
4. Bake in a 350° oven 10-15 minutes or until done.
5. Remove from oven. Slice and serve with baked acorn squash.
6. Drizzle the chicken with sauce from the squash for extra flavor.

PORK TENDERLOIN AND ZITA
Serves 2

10 oz. cooked zita	2 T chopped fresh dill
5 oz. pork tenderloin	½ C chopped scallions
¾ C fat free mayonnaise	¼ C roasted red peppers
½ C fat free sour cream	2 T dijon mustard
¼ C fat free Italian dressing	2 T sweet relish

1. Marinate pork in salad dressing for 30 minutes.
2. Combine remaining ingredients together and mix gently with pasta.
3. Charbroil pork medallions until well done, serve with zita and garnish as desired.

GRILLED SESAME HALIBUT AND LEAF SPINACH
Serves 2

2 - 4 oz. Halibut steaks 1 inch thick	1 tsp. jerk seasoning
1 lb. cleaned and drained leaf spinach	½ C mandarin oranges, drained
½ T sesame seeds	1 C bean sprouts
¼ T olive oil	¼ C julienne red peppers
1 tsp. paprika	½ C fat-free mandarin orange dressing

1. Rub halibut steaks in oil and coat with sesame seeds, paprika and jerk seasoning.
2. Grill quickly on a very hot griddle for 1-2 minutes per side. Remove to a warming dish.
3. Cook halibut in a 350° oven for 3 minutes.
4. Toss spinach with bean sprouts, red peppers, mandarin oranges and dressing. Place on a plate with halibut.
6. Garnish and serve with berry banana delight drink (see recipe).

THE BRAZIEL

Serves 4

4-4 oz. fresh tuna steaks
8 slices high-fiber oatmeal bread

1 package of alfalfa sprouts
8 fresh tomato slices

TUNA MARINADE:

½ T Sesame oil
Juice of 2 limes
Juice of 1 lemon

2 T stone ground mustard
½ C Chardonnay
1 tsp. freshly grated black pepper

1. Marinate tuna steaks for 30-45 minutes, turning one time.
2. Heat non-stick pan or griddle until hot. Place tuna steaks on griddle and cook 3-4 minutes on each side or just until done. Do not overcook as tuna will become dry and tough. It is best cooked medium rare.
3. Spread stone ground mustard on one side of the bread and place tuna on this side. Add alfalfa sprouts and sliced tomatoes.
4. Cut and serve with fruit garnish or your choice of a side dish.

FRUIT GARNISH:

3 strawberries
2 cantaloupe slices

2 oz watermelon
2 oz pineapple

POACHED ATLANTIC SALMON FILLET

Serves 1

1 5oz. boneless salmon fillet
3 oz. peeled, seeded and
   julienne cucumbers

2 oz. yogurt dill sauce (see recipe)
3 oz. shiitake mushrooms - sliced
½ T fresh dill

1. Poach salmon in court bouillon until done 4 - 6 minutes.
2. Place cucumbers in a saute pan and add a little court bouillon to just heat them.
3. Grill shiitake mushrooms on the griddle or in a non-stick pan. Season with fresh dill.
4. Place cucumbers in the middle of the plate with salmon on top of them. Garnish with yogurt dill sauce and sprigs of fresh dill.

HERB BAKED CANADIAN PICKEREL

Serves 1

1 7 oz boneless pickerel fillet
2 T dry bread crumbs
1 tsp. lemon pepper
1 oz. diced onion
1 oz. diced sweet red pepper

1 oz. roma tomato
2 oz. defatted chicken stock
1 C marinara sauce (see sauce section)
½ tsp. olive oil

1. Saute in olive oil the onions, sweet peppers and roma tomatoes until tender. Add chicken stock and marinara sauce. Cook for 5 minutes.
2. Remove from the stove and puree in a blender until smooth. Place back on the stove to simmer until at desired consistency.
3. Combine bread crumbs and lemon pepper seasoning. Dredge pickerel completely and place on silicone paper. Bake in a 350° oven for 10-12 minutes or until done.

4. Remove from the oven. Serve on a heated plate with the reduced sauce. Garnish with grilled zucchini and yellow squash.

CHARBROILED HALIBUT STEAKS WITH CILANTRO CITRUS SAUCE
Serves 2

2 8 oz. halibut steaks, 1 inch thick	2 tsp. fresh chopped cilantro
2 T fat-free lime cilantro dressing	¼ C white wine
Juice of ½ orange	6 tomato slices
Juice of 1 lemon	2 sprigs of fresh cilantro
Juice of 1 lime	2 portions of angel hair pasta

1. Marinate halibut steaks in fat-free lime cilantro dressing for 10-12 minutes.
2. Cook angel hair pasta until tender. Drain but do not rinse.
3. Start charbroiling halibut steaks, about 3 minutes per side. Do not overcook as they will dry out and get tough.
4. Saute angel hair pasta in orange juice, lemon juice, lime juice, white wine and cilantro until hot.
5. Place on a plate with grilled tomato slices and halibut on top of the pasta. Garnish with fresh cilantro.

GRILLED SWORDFISH STEAK
Serves 1

1 5 oz. swordfish steak	1 piece radicchio
2 oz. roasted red pepper	1 tsp. saltless table seasoning
sauce (see recipe)	(see separate recipe)
3 baby corn, grilled	2 cherry tomatoes
1 oz. mesclun greens	1 lemon - juice only

1. Season swordfish with saltless table seasoning. Place on a broiler rack and drizzle with lemon juice.
2. Broil until done on broiler rack (4 - 7 minutes).
3. Place on mesclun greens with radicchio. Ladle roasted red pepper sauce on the greens and plate.
4. Garnish with baby corn and cherry tomatoes.

CREOLE CATFISH
Serves 2

2 6 oz. catfish, farm raised	½ tsp. gumbo file
2 oz. julienne onions	½ C white wine
2 oz. julienne peppers	½ tsp. cayenne pepper
2 oz. sliced mushrooms	1 tsp. olive oil
1 T chopped garlic	2 T flour
1 C marinara sauce	Tabasco sauce - 6 shakes

1. Dredge catfish in flour and saute quickly in non-stick pan with olive oil until just brown.

2. Remove from the pan and place in a shallow baking dish.
3. Place onions, garlic, peppers and mushrooms in the same pan and saute for 3 minutes.
4. Add marinara sauce, gumbo file, white wine, cayenne pepper and Tabasco sauce. Cook for 2 minutes.
5. Add hot mixture over the top of the catfish and bake in the oven for 5 minutes at 350°.
6. Remove from the oven and serve with red beans and rice.

OVEN POACHED SCROD AND WILD GREENS
Serves 2

2-6 oz. boneless and skinless scrod	½ C chardonnay
2 julienne red onions	Juice of 1 lemon
2 oz. julienne zucchini	2 tsp. minced shallots
2 oz. julienne green peppers	½ T chopped parsley
½ T saltless seasoning	2 T fat-free sour cream

1. Place scrod fillets in a shallow baking dish. Season with saltless spices.
2. Put 1/2 mixture of red onions, carrots, zucchini and peppers on each fillet.
3. Squeeze lemon juice on top of the fish.
4. Place white wine in the bottom of the baking dish and cover with aluminum foil. Bake 7-10 minutes at 375°.
5. Remove from the oven and place fish on top of the mixed greens.
6. Add shallots to the liquid and reduce by 1/2. Remove from the heat and whip in sour cream and parsley.
7. Ladle over the fish and serve.

CASHEW CRUSTED ORANGE ROUGHY
Serves 1

7 oz. roughy portion	½ T flour
1 T ground cashews	1 T chopped fresh basil and oregano
1 T dried bread crumbs	

1. In a shallow dish or bowl, combine the cashews, flour and bread crumbs.
2. Season roughy with basil and oregano.
3. Dredge the roughy in the cashew mix and coat completely.
4. Place on a baking pan covered with silicon paper. Sprinkle fish with paprika to get a nice golden brown color. Bake in a 350° oven for 12-15 minutes or until done.
5. Serve with rattatouillie and steamed snow peas.

NORTH CAROLINA GRILLED TROUT
Serves 1

1-8 oz. special boned brook trout	3 oz. fish stock
3 oz. cooked penna pasta	1 oz. shallot raspberry chutney
3 oz. assorted julienne vegetables (leeks, peppers, squash, carrots, snow peas, etc.)	(see sauce section)

MARINADE:

1 C low-sodium tomato juice	1 tsp. onion powder
3 T brown sugar	1 tsp. fresh ground black pepper
1 T molasses	juice of 1 lemon
1 tsp. cayenne pepper	a few drops of liquid smoke
2 tsp. garlic powder	1 T chopped fresh thyme

1. Marinate trout 15-20 minutes or overnight. Heat a non-stick pan and add trout, flesh side down. Cook 1-2 minutes on each side being careful not to overcook. Remove to a hot plate for presentation.
2. Add julienne vegetables to the same pan. Toss around for 1 minute and add fish stock. Add penna pasta and season with fresh thyme.
3. Remove vegetables and pasta mixture from pan and plate with the trout. Serve immediately with shallot raspberry chutney.

GRILLED SHRIMP AND WARM VEGETABLE SALAD CAPELLINI
Serves 4

Two pounds of the following (can substitute any vegetables you like):
white mushrooms

carrots	
bell peppers	1 lb. capellini (angel hair)
yellow squash	1 lb. peeled and deveined shrimp
onion pieces	1 C fat-free lemon herb dressing
broccoli florets	2 T basil
cauliflower	2 T oregano
zucchini	

1. Cut all vegetables into 1-2 inch pieces. Poach or steam until cooked tender. Cool and drain.
2. Marinate chilled vegetables in fat-free lemon herb dressing. Add fresh basil and oregano to the marinade. Amounts depend on your own personal taste. Marinate overnight.
3. Cook pasta until done, rinse in hot water and drain. Place equal amounts on 4 plates and reserve.
4. Cook vegetables on broiler until warm, turning one time to keep from burning. Add some remaining vegetable marinade to the shrimp and place on the griddle or a non-stick pan.
5. Remove vegetables from the broiler and place on top of the pasta. Add shrimp when done.
6. Serve with a side of fat-free dressing.

GRILLED SEA SCALLOPS AND WAX BEANS
Serves 1

1 oz. sea scallops	½ T walnut oil
3 roma tomatoes	3 tsp. rice vinegar
5 oz. yellow and green wax beans	1 tsp. leaf savory
½ T sesame seeds	½ T fat-free italian dressing

1. Marinate scallops in leaf savory and fat-free dressing for 15 minutes.
2. Steam, rinse and drain wax beans. Mix with walnut oil, rice vinegar and sesame seeds.
3. Grill scallops on a non-stick surface until done.
4. Place on a plate with the tomatoes and beans. Drizzle the dressing from the beans on the scallops and tomatoes and garnish as you desire.

TUNA STUFFED BEEFSTEAK TOMATO
Serves 2

8 oz. white meat tuna fish, packed in spring water - drained well
½ C fat-free mayonnaise
¼ C fat-free yogurt
1 T fat-free sour cream
¼ C diced roasted red peppers or pimientos
1 T sweet relish

½ T lemon juice - fresh
1 tsp. stone ground mustard or dijon
2 beefsteak tomatoes
8 oz. romaine lettuce - cut, washed and drained
8 radish roses
6 yellow pepper rings
3 sprigs of opal basil - garnish

1. Mix tuna fish with mayonnaise, yogurt, sour cream, red peppers, sweet relish, mustard and lemon juice.
2. Cut tomatoes from top to bottom onto 6 equal cuts. Be careful not to cut all the way through.
3. Place romaine on a plate with tomato on top. Place 1/2 tuna mixture inside the tomato.
4. Garnish with radish roses, opal basil and yellow pepper rings.
5. Serve with lavish rounds (a fat free dressing of your choice can be added if you choose).

GRILLED SEAFOOD SAUSAGE
Serves 12-14

2 lbs. frozen sole, thawed
½ C egg whites
¼ C diced fresh chives
¼ C diced yellow peppers
¼ C diced green peppers
1 tomato - diced and seeded
1 C cooked baby shrimp

1 tsp. salt
¼ tsp. white pepper
5 shakes Tabasco sauce
2 T chopped parsley
1 T chopped savory
¼ C skim milk

1. Grind sole in a cuisinart or blender with the egg whites and milk until smooth. Remove to a bowl.
2. Add diced chives, yellow peppers, green peppers, tomatoes, shrimp, salt, pepper, parsley and savory.
3. Mix with a spatula until well combined.
4. Roll up into a long tube shape with plastic wrap and tie both ends with string.
5. Poach in 180° water for 45 minutes. Remove to ice cold water to chill.
6. Freeze what you are not going to use.
7. Slice and grill like sausage. Garnish with stone ground mustard and fresh dill.
8. Serve with smoked tomato salsa and marinated white beans.

SEAFOOD RAVIOLI
Makes 48 1/2 oz. ravioli

24 oz. seafood sausage filling
(see recipe)
2 sheets low fat pasta 12 x 12,
any flavor

1 egg white
1 tsp. water

1. Make seafood sausage and chill.
2. Cut sheets to the length and width of the ravioli maker.
3. Place half of the rolled pasta sheet on the bottom of the ravioli maker.
4. Fill each section with 1/2 oz. of seafood sausage mixture.
5. Whip egg white and water until fluffy and brush all edges of the pasta showing.
6. Place other 1/2 of the pasta sheet on top of the ravioli maker and cut with a rolling pin.
7. Repeat this process 3 more times.

RAVIOLI MAKERS CAN BE PURCHASED IN ANY STORE. FOR BEST RESULTS, FOLLOW THE DIRECTIONS FROM THE MANUFACTURER.

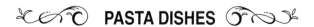 **PASTA DISHES**

PENNA PASTA, HAM AND SNOW PEAS
Serves 2

6 oz. cooked penna
¾ C julienne red onions
¾ C julienne yellow onions
2 T minced elephant garlic
6 oz. of 95% fat-free turkey ham -
julienne

1 C defatted chicken stock
1 T fresh chopped thyme
1 T fresh chopped basil
2 T grated romano cheese
½ T olive oil
1 pkg. julienne snow peas

1. Saute onions, garlic, snow peas and peppers in olive oil until transparent. Add julienne turkey ham and heat.
2. Add chicken stock, thyme and basil. Bring to a boil and add penna.
3. Gently toss, heat completely and remove from heat.
4. Serve with grated romano cheese on top.
5. Garnish with fresh herb of your choice.

ANGEL HAIR WITH PESTO AND GRILLED EGGPLANT
Serves 2

8 oz. cooked angel hair pasta
2 ½ oz. pesto sauce
½ C chopped spinach

6 slices of eggplant - ½ inch thick, no skin
1 T kosher salt
2 T fat-free italian dressing

1. Remove the skin from the eggplant. Place in a glass dish and cover with the salt. Cover with plastic wrap and place in the refrigerator overnight. Turn 2 or 3 times. Remove from the pan and rinse very well. Drain and pat dry. (Step #1 will help the bitter flavors of the eggplant to leach out.)

2. Cook pasta.
3. While the pasta is cooking, brush eggplant with dressing and grill on a non-stick surface for about 2-3 minutes per side.
4. Drain and mix with pesto and spinach.
5. Put pasta in the middle of the plate and arrange cooked eggplant around the pasta.
6. Garnish with fresh basil and cherry tomatoes.

LINGUINI AND JULIENNE VEGETABLES
Serves 2

8 oz. cooked linguini	2 oz. julienne mushrooms
2 oz. julienne onions	18 snow peas cooked and chilled
2 oz. julienne carrots	1 oz. defatted chicken stock
2 oz. julienne peppers	2 T chopped parsley
2 oz. julienne zucchini	1 T butter
2 oz. julienne yellow squash	2 T parmesan cheese
2 tomatoes	

1. Saute tomatoes, onions, carrots, peppers, zucchini, squash and mushrooms in butter until tender.
2. Add cooked linguini, chicken stock and parsley. Cook until all items are hot.
3. Serve on a hot plate with snow peas as a garnish and sprinkle cheese on top.

TOMATO FETTUCCINE WITH MARINARA SAUCE AND ZUCCHINI
Serves 4

1 lb. tomato fettuccine	½ C red wine vinegar
1 lb. crosscut zucchini	4 C marinara sauce (see sauce)
1 T chopped garlic	1 tsp. crushed red pepper
2 T chopped basil	½ C julienne leeks

1. Start cooking fettuccine.
2. Saute garlic and zucchini in a non-stick pan until tender.
3. Add vinegar, marinara sauce, leeks, red pepper and basil. Cover and simmer for 10 minutes.
4. When pasta is done, drain and add the zucchini mix. Toss well and serve on hot platters.
5. Garnish with fresh sprigs of sweet basil.

FARFELLA WITH SWEET BASIL AND LENTILS
Serves 4

8 oz. farfella noodles (large bow ties)	juice of 2 lemons
2 C lentils	1 T chopped basil
2 C defatted chicken stock	½ C chopped scallions
2 T chopped garlic	1 T chopped parsley

1. Cook lentils in chicken stock with garlic until tender.

2. Cook pasta in a separate pot until cooked tender. Remember to not add oil or salt to the water.
3. Drain pasta (do not rinse) and add lemon juice, lentils, scallions, parsley and sweet basil.
4. Toss well and serve.
5. Butter-flavored sprinkles can be added at this point, but remember that they usually contain high levels of sodium, so pick one with low sodium.

PIZZA DOUGH
1 12-inch round

1 package of dry yeast	2 C high gluten flour
1 1/2 tsp granulated sugar	(all purpose can be substituted)
2 T warm water 110°-115°	1 C cold water
1½ tsp. salt	

1. Combine yeast, sugar and warm water in a bowl and let stand in a warm area with no draft for 5 minutes or until very foamy.
2. Combine flour and salt in another bowl and add the yeast mixture while stirring.
3. Mix for 1 minute and add cold water, a little at a time, until all is used up.
4. Place dough on a floured surface and knead for 5 minutes, adding additional flour if necessary.
5. Place dough in a bowl that has been sprayed with fat-free spray and cover the dough completely. Cover with plastic wrap and place in a warm area for 1 hour. (An oven with the pilot light on is a great location.)
6. Dough should double in size. When ready, roll out and make your pizza as desired.

THIS DOUGH CAN BE REFRIGERATED UNTIL THE NEXT DAY.

LOW-FAT PIZZA TOPPING
1 12-inch pizza

8 oz. fat-free ricotta cheese	½ C diced green peppers
4 oz. skim mozzarella	½ C diced green onions
cheese - shredded	1½ C pizza sauce (see recipe below)
½ C diced onion	vegetable spray

1. Saute onions, green peppers and green onions in a non-stick pan with vegetable spray until halfway done.
2. Spread pizza sauce on the pizza dough shell and top with sauteed vegetables. Combine both cheeses in a bowl and sprinkle over the top of the sauce.
3. Bake in a 450° oven until done.

ADDITIONAL TOPPINGS

mushrooms	tuna fish in spring water
fat-free cheese	shrimp
diced tomatoes	chives
smoked salmon	snow peas
(watch sodium amount)	cooked beans

pepperoni	smoked tomato salsa
black olives	breast of chicken
capers	shiitake mushrooms
green olives	lump crabmeat
bean sprouts	napa cabbage
any low-fat cheese of your choice	asparagus
anchovy packed in water	smoked fish of your choice
sardines packed in water	

PIZZA SAUCE
4 Cups

4 C marinara sauce	1 T fresh chopped marjoram
1½ T fresh chopped basil	1 T dried garlic or coarse garlic powder
1½ T fresh chopped oregano	1 C tomato puree

1. Mix all ingredients together cold and use on any pizza of your choice.

RAINBOW ROTINI ALFREDO WITH CHARBROILED VEGETABLES
Serves 2

10 oz. cooked rotini (fusili)	½ C quartered squash
1½ C cream sauce	½ C red peppers
1 C julienne onions	12 mushroom caps
10 asparagus spears	½ C fat-free lemon herb vinaigrette
½ C quartered zucchini	

1. Steam all vegetables and chill quickly. Marinate in fat-free lemon herb vinaigrette.
2. Cook rotini, drain but do not rinse.
3. Heat up cream sauce and pour over the hot rotini and toss gently.
4. Charbroil vegetables to give them flavor.
5. Serve vegetables with rotini and sprinkle grated cheese on top of the pasta.

SPAGHETTI CARBONARA
Serves 4

16 oz. spaghetti, cooked	1 egg
2 tsp. olive oil	2 egg whites
1 T minced shallots	½ cup Parmesan cheese
1 T minced garlic	¼ cup chopped parsley
2 oz. 95% fat free turkey ham julienne	¼ cup skim milk
	½ cup frozen peas, thawed
¼ cup dry white wine	1 tsp. ground black pepper

1. Saute garlic and shallots in olive oil until golden brown but not burnt.
2. Add turkey ham and white wine. Cook for 2 minutes.
3. In a bowl combine eggs, egg whites, cheese, parsley and milk, mix well.
4. Drain spaghetti and place back in the same pot that it was cooked in.
5. Add milk and egg mixture to the pasta while cooking over low heat. Do not over-

cook as it will turn to scrambled eggs.
6. Turn gently while cooking, about 1-1/2 minutes. Remove from the heat, add black pepper and peas, serve.

16

DESSERT RECIPES

At last, desserts, the crowning touch of any meal. Whether shared with friends over conversation, or enjoyed alone lingering over a mocha cappuccino, nothing soothes the soul quite like an elegant dessert.

Chef Edward's desserts are specially designed to be low in fat and calories. So relax, enjoy and treat yourself to one of life's little pleasures. After all, you deserve it since you're eating a new way for a new you!

CHOCOLATE MINT CAROB PUDDING

Serves 8

⅓ C cocoa powder
1 C granulated sugar
1 can evaporated condensed milk
2 C skim milk

¼ C cornstarch
1 tsp. vanilla extract
1 oz carob chips

1. In a sauce pan combine cocoa, sugar, condensed milk, skim milk and cornstarch.
2. Cook over medium heat while stirring constantly. Bring to a boil and cook 1 minute. Remove from heat and cool 10 minutes.
3. Stir in vanilla and mint extract.
4. When mixture is at room temperature, add the carob chips and mix completely. Pour into molded cups and refrigerate.
5. Add sweetened yogurt cheese on top as garnish.

GEORGIA PEACH BEGGARS PURSE

Serves 4

6 Phyllo sheets
4 medium peaches, pitted and
sliced thin
¼ C dried cherries or raisins
2 T pure maple syrup or dark
karo syrup

¼ tsp. cinnamon
¼ tsp. nutmeg
½ T peach brandy
vegetable spray - no fat

1. Combine peaches, cherries, syrup, cinnamon, nutmeg and peach brandy in a bowl. Set aside.
2. Cut Phyllo dough into 4 equal sections.
3. Place 1 sheet on a cutting board and spray with vegetable spray very quickly. Place another Phyllo sheet on top and spray again. Do this for all 6 sheets.
4. Place 1/4 of the filling in the middle and gather up all sides to the middle of the square. Squeeze tightly to make it look like a purse.
5. Place on a baking sheet and cook in a 350° oven for 7-8 minutes or until brown.

SAUTEED PINEAPPLE WITH STRAWBERRY YOGURT SAUCE

1 portion

1 C fresh pineapple - nice slices
¼ C flour
½ tsp. cinnamon
½ C fat-free strawberry yogurt

vegetable spray
fresh mint leaves
carob sprinkles for garnish

1. Dredge pineapple in flour and cinnamon mixture.
2. Heat and spray non stick pan. Saute pineapple until golden brown.
3. Line on a plate and drizzle strawberry yogurt around the pineapple.
4. Garnish with fresh mint and carob sprinkles.

POACHED BARTLETT PEAR AND KIWI BRANDY SAUCE

Serves 2

2 ripe bartlett pears - medium size
4 kiwi - peeled
2 T brandy or cognac

½ T granulated sugar
cocoa - to dust
sprig of mint

1. Poach pear for about 20 minutes or until tender. Let cool in the liquid. This can be done days ahead of time.
2. Puree kiwi in blender until smooth. Add sugar and brandy according to desired taste.
3. Place kiwi sauce on the bottom of the plate and stand up pear in the middle (base needs to be cut) and garnish with cocoa and fresh mint.

POACHING LIQUID

4 C water
½ C granulated sugar
1 T vanilla

½ T lemon juice
1 C white wine

DRIED CHERRY AND ORANGE COOKIES

Makes about 4 doz.

1 C all purpose flour	½ C chopped dried cherries
¾ C wheat flour	¼ C granulated sugar
½ C brown sugar	½ C orange juice
2 tsp. baking powder	¼ C apple sauce
1 tsp. cinnamon	1 egg
¼ tsp. salt	2 T canola oil

1. Combine all ingredients and drop on a ungreased cookie sheet. Bake for 7-10 minutes at 350°.

MAPLE WALNUT RAISIN MUFFINS

Makes 1 doz.

1 C whole wheat flour	½ C egg whites
1½ C all purpose flour	1 T soybean oil
¼ C chopped walnuts	¼ C pure maple syrup
1 tsp. maple walnut extract	¼ C light karo syrup
2 tsp. baking powder	vegetable spray
¼ C shredded carrot	⅔ C skim milk
¼ C shredded zucchini	¼ C raisins

1. In a bowl sift the wheat flour, all purpose flour and baking powder.
2. Combine all the remaining ingredients together and pour over the dry ingredients. Mix completely and scoop into a muffin tin sprayed with the vegetable spray.
3. Bake for 10-12 minutes at 350°.

CHEESE BLINTZES

Makes 8

2 C of fat-free cottage cheese	8 6-inch crepes - store bought, frozen
3 T granulated sugar	2 T fat-free sour cream
½ tsp. vanilla extract	1 T applesauce

1. Using a blender, whip cottage cheese until smooth. Add sugar, vanilla, applesauce and sour cream. Mix completely.
2. Place 1/8 of the mixture in the middle of each crepe and roll up so that all sides are closed and none of the filling can escape.
3. Bake in the oven for 5-6 minutes or until hot and top with any fat-free preserve of your choice. Can even be dusted with cinnamon, powdered sugar or any fresh fruit that is in season.
4. If crepes are difficult to roll, just put them in a hot oven for 30-45 seconds prior to filling.

ANGEL FOOD ALMOND CAKE WITH RASPBERRY COULIS

Makes 24, 1-inch slices

1 C cake flour	1 tsp. almond extract

1¼ C granulated sugar | ¼ tsp. salt
¼ C honey | ¼ tsp. cinnamon
2 C egg whites

1. Sift flour and 1/2 of the sugar.
2. Whip egg whites until foamy and add other 1/2 of the sugar.
3. Add honey, salt, vanilla, almond and cinnamon. Mix well.
4. With a spatula gently fold the sifted flour mixture into the egg white. Mix well but do not overmix.
5. Place in a 12 inch non-stick tube pan and bake for 40-45 minutes at 350° or until golden brown and springs back when done.
6. Remove from the oven and invert. Let cool.
7. Serve with raspberry coulis.

APPLE COBBLER
Serves 6

1 T granulated sugar | ¾ C apple juice
1 T honey | 1 tsp. cinnamon
4 apples, peeled and cored | 1 tsp. nutmeg
½ C apple sauce

1. Combine all of the above ingredients and place in an oven proof pan. Bake for 25 minutes at 350°. Remove from oven.

2 T apple sauce | 2 T 1% milk
½ C oatmeal | ⅛ tsp. salt
½ C all-purpose flour | 1 T honey
2 tsp. Canola oil | 1 T granulated sugar
2 egg whites | 1½ tsp. baking powder

2. Combine all of the remaining ingredients in a bowl and mix well. When apples are removed from the oven, drop mixture over 50% of the apples. Leave room between spoonfuls.
3. Bake for 20 minutes at 350°.
4. Let cool and serve. Can be topped with apple yogurt for additional flavor.

17

BIOTECH GOURMET SAUCES

A n exclusive specialty of the Biotech Method is the use of tasty and nutritious sauces and dips. All of these dips and sauces are low in fat, yet taste great. Feel free to use them as a flavor enhancer on any of the recipes you desire. They're also great by themselves as a dip with fat-free crackers, tortilla chips or other no-fat or low-fat snack foods.

They add little in the way of fat or calories to an entree or dessert, yet they super-power the taste and add much eye appeal. The smoked tomato salsa is great on baked potatoes, while the roasted red pepper sauce goes well with most meat entrees.

Be a bit adventurous and daring. Try these sauces on various foods and in various combinations. That's what makes the Biotech Method so unique — you can customize your food selections to your own individual tastes.

YOGURT CUCUMBER DILL SAUCE
Makes 3 cups

1 C yogurt cheese (see recipe)	½ C fat-free mayonnaise
1 C fat-free sour cream	½ C shredded cucumbers - drained
1½ T fresh dill	Salt to taste
1 T minced shallots	

Combine all ingredients and serve.

SHALLOT RASPBERRY CHUTNEY
Makes 4 cups

2 T chopped shallots
3 C fresh raspberries (or frozen
if necessary)
1 16 oz. jar Major Grey's chutney

1 T granulated sugar
1 T apple cider vinegar
½ T raspberry extract

Combine all ingredients and chill until ready to use.

MARINARA SAUCE
Makes 2½ quarts

2 C chopped onion
2 T chopped garlic
2 cans 22 oz. pear-shaped
peeled tomatoes
1 5 oz. can tomato puree

1 5 oz. can tomato paste
2 C low-sodium tomato juice
1 tsp. ground black pepper
2 T olive oil

1. Saute garlic in olive oil until just turning brown. DO NOT BURN. Add the onions and saute until transparent.
2. While the onions are cooking, drain the pear tomatoes and crush them with your hands.
3. Add tomatoes, juice, puree and paste to the onions and simmer for 1 hour or until desired consistency is reached.
4. Add black pepper. Remove from the heat and chill quickly.

CRANBERRY APPLE RELISH
Makes 2 cups

1 12 oz. can cranberry sauce
1 peeled and diced apple - very fine
1 T shallots - minced

1 T chopped parsley
2 T fresh cranberries - minced (can use
frozen if fresh are not available)

Combine all ingredients and chill until ready to use.

PINEAPPLE CHUTNEY
Makes 1 quart

1 16 oz. jar Major Grey's chutney
1 C pineapple pureed - fresh
½ C raisins

½ C dried cherries
½ C finely chopped green onion

Combine all ingredients and chill well.

SMOKED TOMATO SALSA
Serves 10-12

6 tomatoes skinned,
seeded and diced
1 diced yellow pepper
1 diced green pepper

1 T minced garlic
¼ C diced green onions
2 T chopped parsley
1 T chopped cilantro

1 diced red pepper
1 T minced shallots

salt and white pepper to taste

1. Smoke tomatoes until proper flavor is achieved - about 10-15 minutes.
2. Dice half of the smoked tomatoes and puree remaining tomatoes. Combine both and mix thoroughly. Add remaining ingredients and chill.

SMALL SMOKERS ARE AVAILABLE FOR HOME USE. FOLLOW DIRECTIONS FOR BEST RESULTS.

STRAWBERRY CHEESE
Makes 3 cups

2 C low-fat cream cheese
1 C julienne strawberries

1 T honey
1 T strawberry extract

1. Puree half of the strawberries in a blender until smooth
2. Combine pureed strawberries with the julienne strawberries, strawberry extract, honey and cream cheese. Chill well and serve on toast or bagels in place of high fat items.

CAJUN REMOULADE SAUCE
Serves 6

½ C fat-free mayonnaise
¼ C diced tomatoes
2 T minced green onions
1 T sweet relish
1 T stone ground mustard

3 T fat-free sour cream
½ tsp. chopped capers
¼ tsp. cayenne pepper
1 tsp. worcestershire sauce
salt to taste

1. Combine all ingredients together and chill. This is great over baked potatoes for the extra flavor.

ROASTED GARLIC AND NORTHERN BEAN SPREAD
Makes 2 cups—Use in place of high fat spreads. Can be used for filling with tomatoes, celery or crackers.

2-12 oz. can low-sodium cooked
navy beans or northern beans,
rinsed and drained
4 whole cloves of garlic
vegetable spray
1 T chopped parsley

¼ C diced red onions
¼ C diced yellow peppers
2 T fresh lemon juice
1 tsp. ground black pepper
1 T olive oil
½ C low-sodium tomato juice

1. Put garlic on a baking sheet and spray with vegetable spray very lightly. Place in a 400° oven for 15 minutes. Turn often to prevent burning. Do not burn as it will make the garlic very bitter. Cool.
2. Puree 3/4 of the beans, garlic, olive oil, tomato and lemon juice until smooth.
3. Remove to a bowl and add remaining beans. Stir in well, slightly mashing beans, but leaving them somewhat whole.

4. Add red onions, yellow peppers, parsley, and black pepper. Stir in completely and chill.

ROASTED RED PEPPER SAUCE
Makes 1 quart

2 T chopped shallots
1 lb. can roasted red peppers,
   drained and rinsed (save
   ½ T liquid)
1 C chardonnay

1 T chopped fresh garlic
2 T chopped parsley
½ tsp. white pepper
salt to taste
¼ C skim milk

1. Saute garlic and shallots in liquid saved from the roasted peppers until transparent.
2. Add white wine and reduce by half.
3. Puree red peppers until smooth and add to the white wine mixture.
4. Bring to a boil, add salt, pepper, skim milk and parsley.
5. Remove from stove and chill. Can be reheated at any time. Can also be frozen or kept in the refrigerator for 5-7 days.

BLACK BEAN SAUCE OR DIP
Makes 3 cups

2 C black beans
4 C water
1 C pale dry sherry
1 T ground cumin
1 C orange juice

1 small diced onion
2 T chopped garlic
½ tsp. cayenne pepper
1 tsp. olive oil
Tabasco sauce to taste

1. Soak beans overnight in water. Drain and add 4 cups of water back. Place on the stove to heat up.
2. Saute onions in olive oil with the garlic. Add beans, orange juice, sherry, cumin and cayenne pepper.
3. Cook over medium heat and stir often. When beans are almost done, remove 1/2 of them and puree in a blender. Add back to the original pot and reduce.
4. Can be used as a sauce or dip. Keep that in mind when reducing to the consistency that you desire.

YOGURT CREAM CHEESE
Makes 1 cup

2 C plain non-fat yogurt

1 piece cheese-cloth

1. Line a strainer with cheesecloth and set over a bowl. Add the yogurt and let drain overnight.
2. This can be used in place of cream cheese in a recipe.

PESTO SAUCE
2 cups

8 oz. fresh basil

¼ C fat-free Italian dressing

½ C chopped green onions
4 cloves of garlic

¼ C parmesan cheese
¼ C pine nuts

1. Combine basil, garlic, green onions and pine nuts in a blender. Puree until smooth. Scrape down sides as necessary.
2. With machine running, add dressing and cheese. Remove and use as needed.

PARMESAN AND DILL DIP

Makes about 2 cups

½ C fat-free mayonnaise
½ C non-fat sour cream
½ C fat-free ranch dressing
1 T chopped dill
1 T minced shallots

1 tsp. chopped garlic
1 T stone ground mustard
¼ C parmesan cheese
Tabasco to taste

1. Combine all ingredients in a small bowl and whisk completely. Chill until ready to use.

CREAM SAUCE

Makes about 4 cups

2 C 2% milk
2 C skim milk
¼ C corn starch
3 cloves garlic, chopped

2 T shallots, diced
salt, white pepper to taste
pinch of nutmeg - optional

1. Combine 2% and skim milk. Heat 3 cups of milk with shallots and cloves. Bring to a boil, reduce heat and simmer.
2. Dissolve the cornstarch in remaining cup of milk . Add slowly to the milk. Bring to a boil and cook for 1 minute.
3. Add seasonings to your taste and remove from the heat. Strain and chill quickly.

CAN BE USED AS A BASE FOR ALL CREAM SAUCES.

OVEN ROASTED VEGETABLE MARINARA SAUCE

Makes 1½ quarts

1 quart marinara sauce
1 C onions
1 C yellow squash
1 C zucchini

1 C peppers, red and yellow
4 garlic cloves
1 quart tomatoes
6 green onions

1. Cut all vegetables into 1 inch pieces and place on a cookie sheet or non-stick surface.
2. Place in a 350° oven and roast until golden brown. Be careful to turn often and do not burn.
3. Remove vegetables from the oven and run through a cuisenart or blender until coarse ground. Do not puree totally.
4. Combine with marinara sauce and bring to boil. Let simmer for 10-15 minutes and serve.

RASPBERRY CINNAMON COULIS
Makes 3 Cups

4 C fresh raspberries
¼ cup orange juice
1 T Grenadine
1 T Chambord
½ tsp. cinnamon

1. In a blender combine all ingredients and puree.
2. Set in the refrigerator to chill.

GINGER LIME VINAIGRETTE
Serves 8, makes 1 cup

¼ cup fresh lime juice
1 T minced ginger
¼ tsp. ground coriander
¼ tsp. red pepper flakes
1 T chopped basil
1 T chopped cilantro
1 T lemon juice
½ T chopped parsley
1 T Oyster sauce
1 T Canola oil
1 tsp. sesame oil
salt and pepper to taste

1. Combine all ingredients together except the oil.
2. When ready to serve whisk in the oil and serve over salad greens, chicken or fish for a very tangy topping.

18

SUPERCHARGE FOODS WITH STOCKPOT EXTRACTS, HERBS AND SPICES

C ooking with herbs and spices allows you to use less salt and fat, since the herbs add delightful flavors to foods.

Fresh herbs are usually less flavorful per volume than dried herbs. It is necessary to use more fresh herbs to get the same flavor as with dried herbs. It usually takes double the amount of fresh herbs to get the same taste as with dried herbs.

Store spices in a cool, dry place out of direct sunlight, and use a sealed airtight container. Whole spices stored in this manner retain their natural flavors for long periods of time.

Here are some suggestions for various herbs. The fun of the Biotech Method is that it allows you to experiment and find your favorites. So go ahead, try herbs, and be a little daring. Your taste buds will be delighted.

COMMONLY USED HERBS, SPICES AND FLAVORINGS FOR SUPERCHARGING FOODS WITH FLAVOR:

Bay leaf	Add to soups, potatoes and stews.
Cayenne Pepper	Great for salsa, tacos, chili, chicken and fish.
Chives	Delicate flavored, tall thin leaves from the onion family. Use with eggs and soups.

Cilantro	Also known as fresh coriander. Comes from the parsley family and is pungent in flavor. Used in Oriental, Indian and Spanish cooking.
Cinnamon	Sweet, spicy and mildly pungent in flavor. Used in many dessert preparations.
Cloves	Only small amounts are needed. Use with onion for a good stock.
Cumin/Curry	Use with white meats, pork, yogurt-based dips and rice.
Dill	Mild, pleasing flavor from the parsley family. Used in all types of cooking. Especially good with cucumber salad, potatoes, cottage cheese, rice, salmon, yogurt dips and tomato soup.
Estragon	Good on salads.
Fennel seed	Good with seafood, pork and tomato sauces. (Fennel seed tea is a good tonic for digestive problems, like overeating and indigestion.)
Garlic	Strong pungent flavor. Very versatile and is popular in all types of cooking.
Ginger	Use in stirfry, oriental dishes and salad dressings.
Marjoram	Pleasant flavor, somewhat bitter. Comes from the mint family, and is usually used with poultry, green beans, lamb, seafood and potatoes.
Mint	Perfect with lamb. Add to our appetizer fruit drink recipes to add a bit of zing.
Mustard powder	Great for sauces and dips instead of high-fat oils.
Nutmeg	Seed of nutmeg tree. Warm, highly spicy and is generally used in desserts and baking. Try with bechamel sauce, cheese dishes, fruit salad and vegetable or fruit juice drinks.
Onion	Most widely used, universal seasoning. Member of the lily family. Used in all types of cooking.
Oregano	Strong pungent flavor similar to marjoram. Used in Italian, Greek and Middle Eastern cooking. Good in tomatoes and tomato dishes/sauces and pasta.
Paprika	Good with veal.
Parsley	Mild, pleasant flavored herb that blends well with most foods. Use in salads, soups and potatoes. Also increases the flavor of dried herbs.
Rosemary	Sweet pine-like fragrance. Excellent for marinating lamb, pork and poultry. Perfect for rabbit, lamb, chicken, stews, vegetables and fruit.
Savory	Aromatic flavor from the mint family. Best used in legumes, meat and poultry.
Sweet basil	A pungent clove-like flavor that comes from the mint family. Used in Italian cooking. Use in pasta, salads, chicken, omelets, tomatoes, potatoes, cucumber and squash.
Tarragon	Good for use with salads, fish, chicken and omelets.

Thyme   Slightly pungent, aromatic flavor from the mint family. Excellent in chowders. Also good with lamb, beef, vegetables, soups, fish and rice.

SPICES TO USE WITH VARIOUS TYPES OF FOODS:

Beef - basil, bay leaf, chili pepper, cumin, garlic, ginger, marjoram, onion, oregano, parsley, rosemary, sage, savory, tarragon, thyme.

Chicken - allspice, basil, bay leaf, cinnamon, curry powder, dill, garlic, ginger, marjoram, nutmeg, onion, paprika, parsley, rosemary, saffron, sage, savory, thyme.

Eggs - basil, chervil, chives, coriander, curry powder, dill, fennel, marjoram, oregano, paprika, parsley, rosemary, sage, savory, tarragon, thyme.

Fish - basil, chives, curry powder, dill, garlic, ginger, marjoram, oregano, parsley, sage, savory, tarragon, thyme.

Potatoes - caraway, chives, dill, marjoram, oregano, paprika, parsley, rosemary, tarragon, thyme.

Soups - basil, bay leaf, chives, dill, garlic, marjoram, onion, parsley, rosemary, sage, savory, thyme.

MARINADES FOR SUPERCHARGING FOODS

Marination is used to flavor and tenderize tougher cuts of meat. For poultry or fish, which do not need to be tenderized, using a marinade is your own personal way of adding unique flavors and variety.

The natural acids in marinades break down collagen. This is very important. Collagen is the connective substance in meats which cause it to be tough.

Do not over-marinate tender cuts of beef, or poultry and seafood. This will cause it to become dry, chalky and somewhat mushy.

The following are some examples of items that can be used in marinades. We have included oils which can be used to add flavor but also can be eliminated if so desired.

ACIDS:
Red Wine	White Wine
Cider Vinegar	Tarragon Vinegar
Balsamic Vinegar	Any flavored Vinegars
Lemon Juice	Tomato Juice
Lime Juice	Orange Juice

FOR SWEETNESS:
Dill	Tarragon
Allspice	Cinnamon
Nutmeg	Celery
Carrots	Peppers
Poppyseeds	Anise
Fennel	Orange sections
Pears	Any berries

Nuts	Parsley
Marjoram	

FOR SPICINESS:

Lemon Pepper	Ground Black Pepper
Red Pepper	Tabasco Sauce
Worcestershire Sauce	Cayenne Pepper
Chili Powder	Heinz 57 Sauce
A-1 Steak Sauce	

FOR PUNGENCY:

Rosemary	Thyme
Oregano	Garlic
Onion	Tomatoes
Sesame Seeds - toasted	Basil
Cilantro	Chives
Leaf Savory	

OILS/COMPLEMENTS

Walnut Oil	Olive Oil
Sesame Oil	Peanut Butter
Mayonnaise	Honey
Avocado Oil	Clarified Butter
Peanut Oil	Canola Oil
Chutney	Hazelnut Oil
Almond Oil	Safflower Oil

The beauty of marinades is that there are no rules to what items and how much of anything you can use. Experiment until you find proportions that you like. Eliminate all oils for a fat-free marinade.

Simply mix up several of the ingredients that sound good to you, and marinate the meat for several hours before cooking. You can also marinate beef overnight if you like. (But don't do this to the good, tender cuts. A few hours for the good cuts of beef will do the job.)

Here's the recipe for my Champagne Balsamic Vinaigrette that goes well with vegetables, field greens and pasta salads.

CHAMPAGNE BALSAMIC VINAIGRETTE

1 C champagne	½ tsp. kosher salt
½ C balsamic vinegar	fresh ground black pepper
1 T minced shallots	½ T walnut oil
½ T basil	

1. Combine all ingredients except the oil.
2. When ready to serve, just whisk in the oil at the last minute.

Here are other basic marinades that work well:

QUICK AND EASY MARINADE

3 Cups apple juice
2 Cloves garlic

1 Cup Bragg's Liquid Aminos
(natural soy sauce)

1. Combine all ingredients and pour over food.
2. Let marinate for several hours or longer.

SEAFOOD MARINADE

1 C low sodium tomato juice
3 T brown sugar
1 T molasses
1 tsp. cayenne pepper
2 tsp. garlic powder

1 tsp. onion powder
1 tsp. fresh ground black pepper
juice of 1 lemon
a few drops of liquid smoke
1 T chopped fresh thyme

1. Combine all ingredients and mix well.
2. Marinate fish in the mixture for several hours.

RED WINE HERB VINAIGRETTE

Makes about 4 cups

3 C cabernet saubignon
2 T olive oil
3 shallots, sliced
3 garlic cloves, sliced
1 celery stalk, sliced
1 carrot, sliced
½ T fresh chopped basil

½ T fresh chopped parsley
½ T fresh chopped tarragon
½ T fresh chopped dill
½ T fresh chopped oregano
3 bay leaves
10 black peppercorns

This simple marinade can be used for beef, pork, lamb or chicken. It is a little strong for seafood.

If you wish to use this recipe for seafood, just substitute the cabernet for any dry white wine of your choice and add 1/4 cup of fresh lemon juice.

SUPERCHARGING FOODS WITH FLAVOR — THE STOCKPOT SECRET

The greatest little-known technique that chefs use to boost the flavor of foods is the use of stockpot bases, also known as bouillon, chicken stock and clarified stock.

Several companies make dehydrated stock powders. They are quite easy to use. You simply spoon a teaspoon into a cup of warm water, and voila, instant flavor!

These powdered base stocks come in many flavors and varieties, such as deluxe and premier chicken base, oven-roasted beef and deluxe beef base, beef bouillon, white or red lobster, clam, crab, ham and pork, mushroom, vegetable, shrimp, fish, turkey, veal and lamb bases. Most varieties are available with or without MSG (monosodium glutamate). These powdered base stocks have anywhere from 0 to 1 gram of fat. Some of the commercial powdered stocks are a bit high in sodium. So choose wisely and read the nutrition information label of any powdered stock that you purchase.

By the way, stocks aren't just for making soups. Not with the Biotech Method. We use stocks for sauteing, frying, steaming, poaching, boiling and just about any type of cooking that we do. As an example: Instead of using butter, margarine or oil to saute vegetables, use stock pot base instead. It adds little or no fat, and gives the veggies a delightful flavor. Add some stock base to boiled vegetables, browned meats for fajitas, use when frying special ground meat mix for chili or burgers or whatever else needs to be sauteed.

Because the powders contain salt, I make all my own stocks from scratch. It takes more time, but you can make it all at once and freeze the stock in ice cube trays. Then, as you need stock, simply pop a cube into a pot and you're all set to go! From now on, keep those chicken and turkey carcasses for making your stockpot base. Beef juice drippings can be used for beef-based stocks as well. Here are my favorite stock recipes:

BASIC CHICKEN STOCK
Yield: 1 gallon

2 gallons of cold water	24 parsley stems
5 lbs. chicken rib bones and	12 whole black peppercorns
neck bones	12 whole coriander seeds
1 lb. large cut leeks or onions	6 bay leaves
1 lb. large cut carrots or parsnips	1 T leaf thyme
1 lb. celery	

1. Place bones into a pot and cover with the cold water.
2. Bring to a boil and remove all of the scum that will rise to the top of the pot.
3. Add the remaining ingredients and reduce heat to a slow simmer.
4. Let this cook for 6 hours and remove from the heat.
5. Strain through a sieve into a clean pot and put back onto the heat.
6. Bring back to a simmer and reduce to 1 gallon. Chill stock overnight.
7. When stock is completely chilled, the fat will solidify and can be removed from the top.
8. You now have a very low fat chicken stock.

THIS STOCK CAN BE FROZEN IN QUART JARS OR A GREAT IDEA FOR HOME USE IS TO FREEZE INSIDE ICE CUBE TRAYS SO YOU CAN JUST TAKE OUT A LITTLE AT A TIME. THIS ELIMINATES SPOILAGE AND REDUCES YOUR TIME IN THE KITCHEN.

BASIC BEEF STOCK
Yield: 1 gallon

2 gallons of cold water	1 lb. large cut celery
5 lbs. beef bones, cut	12 whole black peppercorns
1 lb. large cut leeks or onions	6 bay leaves
1 lb. large cut carrots or parsnips	1 T leaf thyme

1. Place bones in a roast pan and into a 350° oven until brown. Turn 2 or 3 times.
2. Add onions, carrots and celery and brown for about 1/2 hour.
3. Remove from the oven, place into a pot and cover with cold water.
4. Add bay leaves, black peppercorns and thyme.
5. Bring to a boil and reduce to a simmer. Cook for 8 hours. Remove from the fire and strain through a sieve into another pot. Place back on the heat, simmer and reduce the stock to 1 gallon.
6. Chill overnight and remove the solidified fat from the top.
7. You now will have low-fat beef stock.

SAME DIRECTIONS AS CHICKEN STOCK FOR FREEZING.

BASIC VEGETABLE STOCK

Yield: 1 gallon

2 gallons cold water	1 leek, washed and large cut
1 medium onion — large cut	12 parsley stems
4 carrots, peeled and large cut	6 bay leaves
4 celery stalks — large cut	12 black peppercorns
4 medium tomatoes	1 tsp. thyme

1. Combine all ingredients and bring to a boil.
2. Reduce heat and let simmer for 45 minutes.
3. Strain and use in place of water or for flavoring foods.

CAN BE FROZEN LIKE CHICKEN STOCK FOR FUTURE USE.

COURT BOUILLON USED FOR POACHING SEAFOOD

2 cups of dry white wine	6 black peppercorns
1 C white vinegar	3 whole cloves
1/2 diced onion	3 bay leaves
2 stalks diced celery	1 tsp. kosher salt or sea salt
1 diced carrot	1 tsp. thyme
12 parsley stems	

1. Combine all ingredients together and bring to a boil. Reduce heat and simmer for 45 minutes.
2. Strain.
3. Poach salmon in this liquid.
4. This liquid can be frozen and reused many times over. It will get a better flavor.

To make your stocks as low in fat as possible, cook them up and chill overnight in the refrigerator. The next day it will be very easy to remove the congealed fat from the stock, as the fat rises to the top and hardens. This way your homemade stock will be low in fat, sodium and calories.

You can also use the following liquids as supercharged flavor stocks: vegetable broth, tomato juice, lemon juice, balsamic vinegar, cooking wine, barbecue sauce or fruit juice. Go ahead and experiment — that's what makes cooking fun.

CUT OUT THE SALT

Salt is non-fattening. Using too much salt, however, does carry a certain amount of health risk, and it may temporarily slow or stop your weight loss.

Using salt may cause or worsen high blood pressure, especially if one is already overweight. Excess weight increases the risk of developing high blood pressure, and salt increases that risk further.

Most of the foods recommended in the Biotech Plan are naturally low in salt. Most often, it's the processed foods or fast food items that are high in sodium content.

Salt also increases water retention in the body, which leaves one feeling bloated and "puffy." Here's why it happens: dietary salt ends up in the various body fluids. Since the body doesn't like salt, water is removed from the cells to try and dilute it. This water goes from the cells into body fluids, which results in the bloated feeling.

Since your cells are now moisture-depleted, you feel thirsty and drink. This excess water then results in a temporary water-weight gain.

So, it would be wise to limit adding salt to your foods. An added benefit is that you'll really begin to enjoy the natural taste of foods without salt. And if you begin using more spices and herbs, unsalted food becomes gourmet-quality and loaded with flavor.

I might add that my Saltless Table Seasoning recipe is quite tasty!

CHEF EDWARD'S SALTLESS TABLE SEASONING

1 T Ground Black Pepper	1 T Dried Basil
2 T Dried Parsley	2 T Coarse Garlic Powder
1 T Dried Marjoram	½ T Cayenne Pepper
1 T Dried Savory	1 T Dried Thyme

1. Put all ingredients into a blender and mix well.
2. Place into a shaker and place on your table instead of salt.
3. Use as often as you like.

NOTE: This recipe can be adjusted however you like for your own personal taste.

TIPS FOR REDUCING SALT IN YOUR MEALS

1. Use fresh herbs instead of salt.
2. Salt can easily be eliminated from any recipe except those containing yeast.
3. Do not add salt to boiling water when cooking pasta.
4. Salty water can be discarded and fresh added when cooking salty foods.
5. Use fresh or frozen foods whenever possible. Avoid using canned foods — they are high in sodium.
6. Reduce consumption of processed lunch meats, bacon, ham, sausage, pickled products, hot dogs or other processed meats.
7. Use fresh meats and specially processed foods that are low in sodium.
8. Avoid recipes that contain baking soda or baking powder. They may contain high levels of sodium.

9. Purchase low sodium crackers, cereals, unsalted margarine and other low or no-salt products.

So there you have it: My secrets on spices, marinades and salt substitutes gathered over a lifetime of gourmet cooking. Use them to impress all your dinner guests, and make them so envious of your new-found cooking skills. One last word of encouragement — be sure to try a good number of the spices, and make several marinades for your favorite meals. Soon you will find just the right combination that suits you the best. The time and effort will be worth it when you taste a low-fat meal that is in every sense of the word a gourmet meal. Again, Bon Appetit!

19

BIOTECH MENU PLANS
FOR WEIGHT LOSS, MUSCLE GAIN
AND WEIGHT MAINTENANCE

T he menu plans that follow are customized using the recipes that appear in this book. They are suggested as a guideline only. Feel free to change them to meet your specific needs. After all, that's what makes the Biotech Method so appealing — you can choose your favorite foods and still lose weight.

You may choose to substitute one type of fish for another more to your liking or you may want to enjoy your main meal of the day at some time other than the customary evening meal time.

Feel free to add snacks as desired. Use Appendix B as a guideline when choosing fat-free snack items.

You may always add steamed vegetables, rice, pasta, salads or potatoes to any entree if you desire more food. Appendix B also lists food selections that you can eat whenever you get hungry. Baked potatoes, wax beans, asparagus, carrots, cauliflower, green beans or broccoli contain less than 1/2 gram of fat per cup, while pasta, baked beans or rice contain only about a gram of fat per cup. These can be added to meals in the menu plan as you desire.

Remember to use sauces and dips as condiments to spice up an entree and add more eye appeal to your meal. Sauces to try include the Smoked Tomato Salsa, Black Bean sauce, Roasted Red Pepper sauce or the Roasted Garlic Spread.

WEIGHT LOSS MENU PLAN
1500 CALORIES PER DAY
(All meals are single servings unless noted otherwise.)

Day 1 Monday

> Breakfast
> Chef Edward's Breakfast #1
>
> Lunch
> Tomato Fettucine with marinara sauce and zucchini
>
> Dinner
> Chicken Almond Stirfry with Herbed Rice Pilaf

Day 2 Tuesday

> Breakfast
> Chef Edward's Breakfast #5
>
> Lunch
> Penna Pasta with ham and snow peas
>
> Dinner
> The Braziel with a cup of Hearty Five Bean soup (1/2 serving)

Day 3 Wednesday

> Breakfast
> Chef Edward's Breakfast #6
>
> Lunch
> Grilled Swordfish Steak with Marinated Asparagus Spears
>
> Dinner
> Turkey Burger with Vegetable Chili

Day 4 Thursday

> Breakfast
> Chef Edward's Breakfast #4
>
> Lunch
> Grilled Tenderloin of Beef and Cous Cous
>
> Dinner
> Grilled Breast of Chicken Palombo with Eggplant Parmesan

Day 5 Friday

> Breakfast
> Chef Edward's Breakfast #5
>
> Lunch
> Angel Hair Pasta and Grilled Eggplant with a Vegetable Kabob (1/2 serving)
>
> Dinner
> Reduced Fat Hamburger and Oven Jerked French Fries

Day 6 Saturday

Breakfast
Chef Edward's Breakfast #3

Lunch
Turkey Parmesan with Oven Roasted Marinara Sauce

Dinner
Grilled Sesame Halibut with spinach (1 1/2 servings)

Day 7 Sunday

Breakfast
Chef Edward's Breakfast #6

Lunch
Grilled Vegetarian Sandwich with Polenta Mushrooms

Dinner
Grilled Boneless Breast of Chicken with Pineapple Chutney

Day 8 Monday

Breakfast
Chef Edward's Breakfast #4

Lunch
Pepper Steak Barley Soup with Julienne Vegetable Chow Mein

Dinner
Farfella with Lentils and Sweet Basil

Day 9 Tuesday

Breakfast
Chef Edward's Breakfast #8

Lunch
North Carolina Grilled Trout (1/2 serving)

Dinner
Cous Cous and Grilled Onion Hamburger with Spicy Napa Cole Slaw

Day 10 Wednesday

Breakfast
Chef Edward's Breakfast #5

Lunch
Shrimp and Barley Salad (1/2 serving)

Dinner
2 servings of Turkey Meatloaf with 1/2 serving of Red Bliss Potatoes

Day 11 Thursday

Breakfast
Chef Edward's Breakfast #7

Lunch
Pork Tenderloin and Zita (1/2 serving)
Dinner
Oven Fried Chicken Breast with a Twice Baked Potato

Day 12 *Friday*

Breakfast
Chef Edward's Breakfast #4
Lunch
Rainbow Rotini Alfredo with Charbroiled Vegetables
Dinner
Oven Poached Scrod with wild greens and a serving of Red Beans and Rice

Day 13 *Saturday*

Breakfast
Chef Edward's Breakfast #2
Lunch
Low-fat Pizza with Chef Edward's special topping, sauce and dough
Dinner
Poached Breast of Chicken (1 1/2 servings)

Day 14 *Sunday*

Breakfast
Chef Edward's Breakfast #1
Lunch
Beef Medallions & Jicama (1/2 serving)
Dinner
Linguini and Julienne Vegetables

Day 15 *Monday*

Breakfast
Chef Edward's Breakfast #1
Lunch
Tomato Fettucine with marinara sauce and zucchini
Dinner
Chicken Almond Stirfry with Herbed Rice Pilaf

Day 16 *Tuesday*

Breakfast
Chef Edward's Breakfast #5
Lunch
Penna Pasta with ham and snow peas
Dinner
The Braziel with a cup of Hearty Five Bean soup (1/2 serving)

Day 17 Wednesday

Breakfast
Chef Edward's Breakfast #6

Lunch
Grilled Swordfish Steak with Marinated Asparagus Spears

Dinner
Turkey Burger with Vegetable Chili

Day 18 Thursday

Breakfast
Chef Edward's Breakfast #4

Lunch
Grilled Tenderloin of Beef and Cous Cous

Dinner
Grilled Breast of Chicken Palombo with Eggplant Parmesan

Day 19 Friday

Breakfast
Chef Edward's Breakfast #5

Lunch
Angel Hair Pasta and Grilled Eggplant with a Vegetable Kabob (1/2 serving)

Dinner
Reduced Fat Hamburger and Oven Jerked French Fries

Day 20 Saturday

Breakfast
Chef Edward's Breakfast #3

Lunch
Turkey Parmesan with Oven Roasted Marinara Sauce

Dinner
Grilled Sesame Halibut with spinach (1 1/2 servings)

Day 21 Sunday

Breakfast
Chef Edward's Breakfast #6

Lunch
Grilled Vegetarian Sandwich with Polenta Mushrooms

Dinner
Grilled Boneless Breast of Chicken with Pineapple Chutney

Day 22 Monday

Breakfast
Chef Edward's Breakfast #4

Lunch
Pepper Steak Barley Soup with Julienne Vegetable Chow Mein
Dinner
Farfella with Lentils and Sweet Basil

Day 23 *Tuesday*

Breakfast
Chef Edward's Breakfast #8

Lunch
North Carolina Grilled Trout (1/2 serving)

Dinner
Cous Cous and Grilled Onion Hamburger with Spicy Napa Cole Slaw

Day 24 *Wednesday*

Breakfast
Chef Edward's Breakfast #5

Lunch
Shrimp and Barley Salad (1/2 serving)

Dinner
2 servings of Turkey Meatloaf with 1/2 serving of Red Bliss Potatoes

Day 25 *Thursday*

Breakfast
Chef Edward's Breakfast #7

Lunch
Pork Tenderloin and Zita (1/2 serving)

Dinner
Oven Fried Chicken Breast with a Twice Baked Potato

Day 26 *Friday*

Breakfast
Chef Edward's Breakfast #4

Lunch
Rainbow Rotini Alfredo with Charbroiled Vegetables

Dinner
Oven Poached Scrod with wild greens and a serving of Red Beans and Rice

Day 27 *Saturday*

Breakfast
Chef Edward's Breakfast #2

Lunch
Low-fat Pizza with Chef Edward's special topping, sauce and dough

Dinner
Poached Breast of Chicken (1 1/2 servings)

Day 28 Sunday

Breakfast
Chef Edward's Breakfast #1

Lunch
Beef Medallions & Jicama (1/2 serving)

Dinner
Linguini and Julienne Vegetables

WEIGHT MAINTENANCE MENU PLAN
2000 CALORIES PER DAY
(All meals are single servings unless noted otherwise.)

Day 1 Monday

Breakfast
Chef Edward's Breakfast #4

Lunch
Tomato Fettucine with marinara sauce and zucchini (1 1/2 servings)

Dinner
Chicken Almond Stirfry with Herbed Rice Pilaf

Day 2 Tuesday

Breakfast
Chef Edward's Breakfast #1

Lunch
Penna Pasta with ham and snow peas (1 1/2 servings)

Dinner
The Braziel with a cup of Hearty Five Bean soup

Day 3 Wednesday

Breakfast
Chef Edward's Breakfast #3

Lunch
Grilled Swordfish Steak with Marinated Asparagus Spears (1 1/2 servings)

Dinner
Turkey Burger with Vegetable Chili

Day 4 Thursday

Breakfast
Chef Edward's Breakfast #6

Lunch
Grilled Tenderloin of Beef and Cous Cous (1 1/2 servings)

Dinner
Grilled Breast of Chicken Palombo with Eggplant Parmesan (1 1/2 servings)

Day 5 *Friday*

Breakfast
Chef Edward's Breakfast #4
Lunch
Angel Hair Pasta and Grilled Eggplant with a Vegetable Kabob
Dinner
Reduced Fat Hamburger and Oven Jerked French Fries (1 1/2 servings)

Day 6 *Saturday*

Breakfast
Chef Edward's Breakfast #2
Lunch
Turkey Parmesan with Oven Roasted Marinara Sauce (1 1/2 servings)
Dinner
Grilled Sesame Halibut with spinach (2 servings)

Day 7 *Sunday*

Breakfast
Chef Edward's Breakfast #8
Lunch
Grilled Vegetarian Sandwich with Polenta Mushrooms
Dinner
Grilled Boneless Breast of Chicken with Pineapple Chutney
(2 servings)

Day 8 *Monday*

Breakfast
Chef Edward's Breakfast #6
Lunch
Pepper Steak Barley Soup with Julienne Vegetable Chow Mein
Dinner
Farfella with Lentils and Sweet Basil (2 servings)

Day 9 *Tuesday*

Breakfast
Chef Edward's Breakfast #5
Lunch
North Carolina Grilled Trout
Dinner
Cous Cous and Grilled Onion Hamburger with Spicy Napa Cole Slaw

Day 10 Wednesday

Breakfast
Chef Edward's Breakfast #7

Lunch
Shrimp and Barley Salad (1/2 serving)

Dinner
Turkey Meatloaf with Red Bliss Potatoes (2 servings)

Day 11 Thursday

Breakfast
Chef Edward's Breakfast #8

Lunch
Pork Tenderloin and Zita

Dinner
Oven Fried Chicken Breast with a Twice Baked Potato (2 servings)

Day 12 Friday

Breakfast
Chef Edward's Breakfast #2

Lunch
Rainbow Rotini Alfredo with Charbroiled Vegetables

Dinner
Oven Poached Scrod with wild greens and a serving of Red Beans and Rice

Day 13 Saturday

Breakfast
Chef Edward's Breakfast #3

Lunch
Low-fat Pizza with Chef Edward's special topping, sauce and dough
(2 servings)

Dinner
Poached Breast of Chicken (2 servings)

Day 14 Sunday

Breakfast
Chef Edward's Breakfast #4

Lunch
Beef Medallions & Jicama

Dinner
Linguini and Julienne Vegetables

Day 15 Monday

Breakfast
Chef Edward's Breakfast #4

Lunch
Tomato Fettucine with marinara sauce and zucchini (1 1/2 servings)
Dinner
Chicken Almond Stirfry with Herbed Rice Pilaf

Day 16 Tuesday

Breakfast
Chef Edward's Breakfast #1
Lunch
Penna Pasta with ham and snow peas (1 1/2 servings)
Dinner
The Braziel with a cup of Hearty Five Bean soup

Day 17 Wednesday

Breakfast
Chef Edward's Breakfast #3
Lunch
Grilled Swordfish Steak with Marinated Asparagus Spears (1 1/2 servings)
Dinner
Turkey Burger with Vegetable Chili

Day 18 Thursday

Breakfast
Chef Edward's Breakfast #6
Lunch
Grilled Tenderloin of Beef and Cous Cous (1 1/2 servings)
Dinner
Grilled Breast of Chicken Palombo with Eggplant Parmesan (1 1/2 servings)

Day 19 Friday

Breakfast
Chef Edward's Breakfast #4
Lunch
Angel Hair Pasta and Grilled Eggplant with a Vegetable Kabob
Dinner
Reduced Fat Hamburger and Oven Jerked French Fries (1 1/2 servings)

Day 20 Saturday

Breakfast
Chef Edward's Breakfast #2
Lunch
Turkey Parmesan with Oven Roasted Marinara Sauce (1 1/2 servings)
Dinner
Grilled Sesame Halibut with spinach (2 servings)

Day 21 Sunday

Breakfast
Chef Edward's Breakfast #8

Lunch
Grilled Vegetarian Sandwich with Polenta Mushrooms

Dinner
Grilled Boneless Breast of Chicken with Pineapple Chutney
(2 servings)

Day 22 Monday

Breakfast
Chef Edward's Breakfast #6

Lunch
Pepper Steak Barley Soup with Julienne Vegetable Chow Mein

Dinner
Farfella with Lentils and Sweet Basil (2 servings)

Day 23 Tuesday

Breakfast
Chef Edward's Breakfast #5

Lunch
North Carolina Grilled Trout

Dinner
Cous Cous and Grilled Onion Hamburger with Spicy Napa Cole Slaw

Day 24 Wednesday

Breakfast
Chef Edward's Breakfast #7

Lunch
Shrimp and Barley Salad (1/2 serving)

Dinner
Turkey Meatloaf with Red Bliss Potatoes (2 servings)

Day 25 Thursday

Breakfast
Chef Edward's Breakfast #8

Lunch
Pork Tenderloin and Zita

Dinner
Oven Fried Chicken Breast with a Twice Baked Potato (2 servings)

Day 26 Friday

Breakfast
Chef Edward's Breakfast #2

Lunch
Rainbow Rotini Alfredo with Charbroiled Vegetables

Dinner
Oven Poached Scrod with wild greens and a serving of Red Beans and Rice

Day 27 Saturday

Breakfast
Chef Edward's Breakfast #3

Lunch
Low-fat Pizza with Chef Edward's special topping, sauce and dough
(2 servings)

Dinner
Poached Breast of Chicken (2 servings)

Day 28 Sunday

Breakfast
Chef Edward's Breakfast #4

Lunch
Beef Medallions & Jicama

Dinner
Linguini and Julienne Vegetables

MUSCLE GAIN MENU PLAN
2500 CALORIES PER DAY
(All meals are single servings unless noted otherwise.)

Day 1 Monday

Breakfast
Chef Edward's Breakfast #6

Lunch
Tomato Fettucine with marinara sauce and zucchini (2 servings)

Dinner
Chicken Almond Stirfry with Herbed Rice Pilaf (1 1/2 servings)

Day 2 Tuesday

Breakfast
Chef Edward's Breakfast #8

Lunch
Penna Pasta with ham and snow peas (2 servings)

Dinner
The Braziel with a cup of Hearty Five Bean soup

Day 3 Wednesday

    Breakfast
    Chef Edward's Breakfast #2

    Lunch
    Grilled Swordfish Steak with Marinated Asparagus Spears (2 servings)

    Dinner
    Turkey Burger with Vegetable Chili

Day 4 Thursday

    Breakfast
    Chef Edward's Breakfast #7

    Lunch
    Grilled Tenderloin of Beef and Cous Cous (2 servings)

    Dinner
    Grilled Breast of Chicken Palombo with Eggplant Parmesan (2 servings)

Day 5 Friday

    Breakfast
    Chef Edward's Breakfast #1

    Lunch
    Angel Hair Pasta and Grilled Eggplant with a Vegetable Kabob (1 1/2 servings)

    Dinner
    Reduced Fat Hamburger and Oven Jerked French Fries (1 1/2 servings)

Day 6 Saturday

    Breakfast
    Chef Edward's Breakfast #8

    Lunch
    Turkey Parmesan with Oven Roasted Marinara Sauce (2 servings)

    Dinner
    Grilled Sesame Halibut with spinach (3 servings)

Day 7 Sunday

    Breakfast
    Chef Edward's Breakfast #2

    Lunch
    Grilled Vegetarian Sandwich with Polenta Mushrooms (1 1/2 servings)

    Dinner
    Grilled Boneless Breast of Chicken with Pineapple Chutney (2 servings)

Day 8 Monday

    Breakfast
    Chef Edward's Breakfast #1

Lunch
Pepper Steak Barley Soup with Julienne Vegetable Chow Mein
(1 1/2 servings)
Dinner
Farfella with Lentils and Sweet Basil and Braised Fennel (2 servings)

Day 9 Tuesday

Breakfast
Chef Edward's Breakfast #7
Lunch
North Carolina Grilled Trout
Dinner
Cous Cous and Grilled Onion Hamburger with Spicy Napa Cole Slaw
(1 1/2 servings)

Day 10 Wednesday

Breakfast
Chef Edward's Breakfast #8
Lunch
Shrimp and Barley Salad
Dinner
Turkey Meatloaf with Red Bliss Potatoes (3 servings)

Day 11 Thursday

Breakfast
Chef Edward's Breakfast #6
Lunch
Pork Tenderloin and Zita (1 1/2 servings)
Dinner
Oven Fried Chicken Breast with a Twice Baked Potato (3 servings)

Day 12 Friday

Breakfast
Chef Edward's Breakfast #2
Lunch
Rainbow Rotini Alfredo with Charbroiled Vegetables (1 1/2 servings)
Dinner
Oven Poached Scrod with wild greens and a serving of Red Beans and Rice
(2 servings)

Day 13 Saturday

Breakfast
Chef Edward's Breakfast #5
Lunch
Low-fat Pizza with Chef Edward's special topping, sauce and dough (3 servings)

Dinner
Poached Breast of Chicken (2 1/2 servings)

Day 14 Sunday

Breakfast
Chef Edward's Breakfast #1

Lunch
Beef Medallions & Jicama

Dinner
Linguini and Julienne Vegetables (2 servings)

Day 15 Monday

Breakfast
Chef Edward's Breakfast #6

Lunch
Tomato Fettucine with marinara sauce and zucchini (2 servings)

Dinner
Chicken Almond Stirfry with Herbed Rice Pilaf (1 1/2 servings)

Day 16 Tuesday

Breakfast
Chef Edward's Breakfast #8

Lunch
Penna Pasta with ham and snow peas (2 servings)

Dinner
The Braziel with a cup of Hearty Five Bean soup

Day 17 Wednesday

Breakfast
Chef Edward's Breakfast #2

Lunch
Grilled Swordfish Steak with Marinated Asparagus Spears (2 servings)

Dinner
Turkey Burger with Vegetable Chili

Day 18 Thursday

Breakfast
Chef Edward's Breakfast #7

Lunch
Grilled Tenderloin of Beef and Cous Cous (2 servings)

Dinner
Grilled Breast of Chicken Palombo with Eggplant Parmesan (2 servings)

Day 19 Friday

Breakfast
Chef Edward's Breakfast #1

Lunch
Angel Hair Pasta and Grilled Eggplant with a Vegetable Kabob
(1 1/2 servings)

Dinner
Reduced Fat Hamburger and Oven Jerked French Fries (1 1/2 servings)

Day 20 Saturday

Breakfast
Chef Edward's Breakfast #8

Lunch
Turkey Parmesan with Oven Roasted Marinara Sauce (2 servings)

Dinner
Grilled Sesame Halibut with spinach (3 servings)

Day 21 Sunday

Breakfast
Chef Edward's Breakfast #2

Lunch
Grilled Vegetarian Sandwich with Polenta Mushrooms (1 1/2 servings)

Dinner
Grilled Boneless Breast of Chicken with Pineapple Chutney (2 servings)

Day 22 Monday

Breakfast
Chef Edward's Breakfast #1

Lunch
Pepper Steak Barley Soup with Julienne Vegetable Chow Mein
(1 1/2 servings)

Dinner
Farfella with Lentils and Sweet Basil and Braised Fennel (2 servings)

Day 23 Tuesday

Breakfast
Chef Edward's Breakfast #7

Lunch
North Carolina Grilled Trout

Dinner
CousCous and Grilled Onion Hamburger with Spicy Napa Cole Slaw
(1 1/2 servings)

Day 24 Wednesday

Breakfast
Chef Edward's Breakfast #8

Lunch
Shrimp and Barley Salad

Dinner
Turkey Meatloaf with Red Bliss Potatoes (3 servings)

Day 25 Thursday

Breakfast
Chef Edward's Breakfast #6

Lunch
Pork Tenderloin and Zita (1 1/2 servings)

Dinner
Oven Fried Chicken Breast with a Twice Baked Potato (3 servings)

Day 26 Friday

Breakfast
Chef Edward's Breakfast #2

Lunch
Rainbow Rotini Alfredo with Charbroiled Vegetables (1 1/2 servings)

Dinner
Oven Poached Scrod with wild greens and a serving of Red Beans and Rice
(2 servings)

Day 27 Saturday

Breakfast
Chef Edward's Breakfast #5

Lunch
Low-fat Pizza with Chef Edward's special topping, sauce and dough
(3 servings)

Dinner
Poached Breast of Chicken 2 1/2 servings)

Day 28 Sunday

Breakfast
Chef Edward's Breakfast #1

Lunch
Beef Medallions & Jicama

Dinner
Linguini and Julienne Vegetables (2 servings)

CHEF EDWARD'S BREAKFAST MENUS

Here are the breakfast recipes used in the Biotech food plans. We've rotated them among the various days in the plan so as to give good variety in your morning meals. Feel free to change or rotate them however you like to fit in with your particular eating plan.

Breakfast #1

1 C dry cereal
½ skim milk
½ C orange juice
1 C strawberries
¼ C non fat flavored yogurt
Hot beverage of your choice

Breakfast #2

1 C Hot oatmeal with cinnamon and
   dried raisins
1 fat-free spice muffin
1 T preserves
½ cantaloupe
¼ C fat-free cottage cheese
Hot beverage of your choice

Breakfast #3

1 C scrambled egg substitute with
   peppers and onions
2 pieces of whole wheat toast
2 T honey
1 C grapefruit juice
1 C skim milk
Hot beverage of your choice

Breakfast #4

1 poached egg on buckwheat pancake
3 oz. grilled mushrooms
1 C tomato juice with celery stick
   garnish
1 C honey dew
¼ C strawberry fat-free yogurt
Hot beverage of your choice

Breakfast #5

1 C cold cereal of your choice
½ C skim milk
½ whole wheat bagel
2 oz. fat-free cream cheese with
   fresh chives
1 oz. raspberry jam
1 C orange juice
Hot beverage of your choice

Breakfast #6

2 banana pancakes with apple butter
1 C fresh blueberries
1 C fat-free yogurt, any flavor
1 oz. orange marmalade
Hot beverage of your choice

Breakfast #8

2 cheese blintzes with strawberry
   yogurt
1 C sliced kiwi fruit
1 fresh baked fat-free muffin
1 piece of whole wheat toast
1 C skim milk
Hot beverage of your choice

Breakfast #7

1 scrambled egg substitute with
   part skim mozzarella cheese
2 oz. 95% turkey ham - grilled
1 bagel - grilled
2 oz. fat-free cream cheese
1 C grape juice
Hot beverage of your choice

20

DINING OUT THE BIOTECH WAY

Cutting down on fat intake doesn't mean that you can't eat out — either in your favorite "white tablecloth" establishment, or at the local fast food restaurant.

Throughout this book, you've been given hints, tips, recipes and ideas on how to cut down on your fat intake. Most of those tips easily apply to dining out in your favorite sit-down restaurant. Remember — ask to have your food boiled, broiled or poached without oils instead of sauted, deep-fat fried or topped with butter or other high-fat sauces. Stick to salads, vegetables, complex carbohydrates and small portions of protein foods.

For your convenience, we've prepared the following chart to help you eat low-fat when you dine out.

HOW GOOD ARE FAST FOODS, AKA "JUNK FOODS"?

Today, it is rare to find a community without a conglomeration of fast food establishments. A recent Gallup survey found that 42% of meals were eaten away from home, with Americans spending $43 billion on the fast food segment.

It was only ten years ago that the expression "junk food" became a part of our vocabulary. Foods cited as "junk" traditionally include pizza, candy, hamburgers, french fries, milkshakes, soft drinks, etc.

Fast foods are typically high in sugar, fat, calories and salt. Rarely is it

```
┌─────────────────────────────────────────────────────────────┐
│              TIPS TO DINING OUT IN RESTAURANTS               │
│                                                             │
│   1.  Choose seafood, poultry and lean meat.                │
│                                                             │
│   2.  Watch for processed foods.  They are usually high in  │
│       fat content.                                          │
│                                                             │
│   3.  Choose low-fat or fat-free yogurts.                   │
│                                                             │
│   4.  Ask what type of oil, if any, is used for cooking.    │
│                                                             │
│   5.  Request skim milk if it's available.                  │
│                                                             │
│   6.  Limit consumption of processed cheese foods.  Ask     │
│       for low-fat cottage cheese or cheese made with part   │
│       skim milk.                                            │
│                                                             │
│   7.  Choose more fruits, vegetables and grains instead of  │
│       foods high in fat content.                            │
│                                                             │
│   8.  Order fat-free or low-fat salad dressings.            │
│                                                             │
│   9.  Use condiments such as mustard, chutneys or relish-   │
│       es instead of mayonnaise.                             │
│                                                             │
│  10.  Eliminate fried foods.  Ask for your foods to be      │
│       poached or broiled.  Do not be intimidated.  You're   │
│       the customer, so ask for what you want.               │
│                                                             │
│  11.  Ask if there is a special low-fat menu.               │
│                                                             │
│  12.  Order all sauces and dressings, if any, on the side.  │
│                                                             │
│  13.  Avoid baked goods made with palm oil, coconut oil or  │
│       lard.                                                 │
│                                                             │
│  14.  If ordering any meat, request that all visible fat be cut │
│       off your portion prior to cooking.                    │
│                                                             │
│  15.  Avoid butter, sauted, fried or crispy foods, hol-     │
│       landaise sauces, casseroles, escalloped, augratin,    │
│       stewed or pan-fried foods.                            │
│                                                             │
└─────────────────────────────────────────────────────────────┘
```

mentioned that fast food refers to the way in which food is prepared, as well as the speed with which it is served.

Opinions on what foods are "junk" vary. Whether you consider a food nutritious or "junk" probably lies within the context of the rest of your diet. That is to say, the total diet, not the individual foods, should be assessed. Any food can find its place in the diet with proper nutrition education. Yes, even the occasional splurge of a burger and fries can be handled by your body if you eat well the rest of the time.

The fast food industry has been responsive to consumer interest in the nutritive value of its foods. Many of the fast food chains now provide nutrient analyses of their foods. As an example, consumers said they wanted more chicken and fish and less beef. Fast food chains were delighted. After all, chicken and fish are cheaper than beef. The problem lies in the fact that most of these new chicken and fish dishes come battered, breaded and deep-fat fried, making them high in fat content.

On the other hand, salad bars are now available at many of the chains. But remember — if you eat your salad with a high-fat dressing, you may have defeated your purpose. (One ladle of fat-based dressing can add 200 calories or more.)

The bottom line for good nutrition rests with the consumer. Fast foods are still food, and no food should be considered totally worthless. True, some are of limited nutritional value, but better food choices, both at home and away from home, are the answer.

Eating low-fat at the local fast food restaurant requires a bit more work. You usually cannot specify changes in the menu or the cooking method. And many of us at least occasionally eat fast food due to our hectic lifestyles. Thankfully, many fast food restaurants are now providing lower calorie foods, some low-fat cooking methods, as well as detailed nutritional information on their products.

It is possible to eat a relatively low-fat meal at a fast food restaurant. Here are tips that we've found to be the most important:

- Augment a fast food sandwich with fruit, salads or vegetables.

- Watch out for batter-fried foods — they're loaded with fat.

- Skip the fat-laden special sauces and toppings. Stay with mustard and ketchup instead.

- Say "NO" to greasy french fries - get a healthy side dish instead. Many restaurants now offer a variety of salads, cole slaw, vegetables, rice, baked potatoes and other foods which are low in fat.

To help you make educated food choices, we've included the following guide to help you eat the Biotech Low-Fat Way even in fast food restaurants. Enjoy!

Arby's

	Calories	FAT gm	Sodium gm
Entrees			
Beef 'n Cheddar (7 oz.)	455	27	955
Junior Roast Beef (3 oz.)	218	8	345
King Roast Beef (6.75 oz.)	467	19	766
Regular Roast Beef (5.2 oz.)	353	15	588
Super Roast Beef (8.25 oz.)	501	22	798

Burger King

	Calories	FAT gm	Sodium gm
Breakfast Items			
Breakfast Bagel Sandwich	387	14	780
Breakfast Bagel Sandwich with Bacon	438	19	905
Breakfast Bagel Sandwich with Ham	418	15	1130
Breakfast Bagel Sandwich with Sausage	621	36	1185
Breakfast Croissanwich	304	19	637
Breakfast Croissanwich with Bacon	355	24	762

Burger King (continued)

	Calories	FAT gm	Sodium gm
Breakfast Croissanwich with Ham	335	20	987
Breakfast Croissanwich with Sausage	538	41	1042
French Toast Sticks	499	29	498
Great Danish	500	36	288
Scrambled Egg Platter	468	30	808
Scrambled Egg Platter with Bacon	536	36	975
Scrambled Egg Platter with Sausage	702	52	1213
Entrees			
Bacon Double Cheeseburger	510	31	728
Cheeseburger	317	15	651
Chicken Specialty Sandwich	688	40	1423
Chicken Tenders (6 pieces)	204	10	636
Ham & Cheese Specialty Sandwich	471	23	1534
Hamburger	275	12	509
"Whaler"	488	27	592
"Whopper"	628	36	880
"Whopper" with Cheese	711	43	1164
Whopper Junior	322	17	486
Whopper Junior with Cheese	364	20	628
Side Dishes			
French Fries, Regular	227	13	160
Onion Rings, Regular	274	16	665
Desserts			
Apple Pie	305	12	412
Beverages			
Coffee, (regular)	2	0	2
Diet Pepsi®, (regular)	1	0	*
Milk, 2% Lowfat	121	5	122
Milk, Whole	157	9	119
Orange Juice	82	0	2
Pepsi Cola®, (regular)	159	0	*
7up®	144	0	*
Shake, Chocolate Medium	320	12	202
Shake, Vanilla Medium	321	10	205
Salads			
Chef Salad	180	9	570
Chicken Salad	140	4	440
Garden Salad	90	5	125
Side Salad	20	0	20
Toppings (packets)			
Bacon Bits	16	1	1
Bleu Cheese dressing	300	31	600
Croutons	29	1	88
French dressing	280	23	690
House dressing	260	26	530
1000 Island dressing	240	23	470
Reduced Calorie Italian dressing	30	2	870

* Indicates that information for this nutrient has not been analyzed or is not available.

Domino's Pizza

Entrees	Calories	FAT gm	Sodium gm
Cheese Pizza, Large (16"), 2 slices	376	10	483
Deluxe Pizza, Large (16"), 2 slices	498	20	954
Double Cheese/Pepperoni Pizza, Large (16"), 2 slices	545	25	1042
Ham Pizza, Large (16"), 2 slices	417	11	805
Pepperoni Pizza, Large (16"), 2 slices	460	18	825
Sausage/Mushroom Pizza, Large (16"), 2 slices	430	16	552
Veggie Pizza, Large (16"), 2 slices	498	19	1035

Kentucky Fried Chicken

	Calories	FAT gm	Sodium gm
Entrees			
"Chicken Littles" Sandwich	169	10	331
Extra Crispy Chicken			
Center Breast	353	21	842
Drumstick	173	11	346
Side Breast	354	24	797
Thigh	371	26	766
Wing	218	16	437
Original Recipe Chicken			
Center Breast	283	15	672
Drumstick	146	8	275
Side Breast	267	16	735
Thigh	294	20	619
Wing	178	12	372
"Kentucky Nuggets" 6 pieces	276	17	840
"Kentucky Nuggets" Sauces			
Barbeque	35	<1	450
Honey	49	<1	<15
Mustard	36	<1	346
Sweet and Sour	58	<1	148
Side Dishes			
Buttermilk Biscuit	232	12	539
Cole Slaw	119	7	197
Corn-on-the Cob	176	3	<21
French Fries, (regular)	244	12	139
Mashed Potatoes with Gravy	71	2	342

McDonald's

	Calories	FAT gm	Sodium gm
Breakfast Items			
Biscuit with spread	260	13	730
Biscuit with Bacon, Egg & Cheese	440	26	1230
Biscuit with Sausage	440	29	1080
Biscuit with Sausage & Egg	520	34	1250
Danish, Apple	390	18	370
Danish, Cinnamon Raisin	440	21	430

McDonald's (continued)

	Calories	FAT gm	Sodium gm
Danish, Iced Cheese	390	22	420
Danish, Raspberry	410	16	310
"Egg McMuffin"	290	11	740
English Muffin with Butter	170	5	270
Hash Brown Potatoes	130	7	330
Hot Cakes with Butter, Syrup	410	9	640
Pork Sausage	180	16	350
"Sausage McMuffin"	370	22	830
"Sausage McMuffin" with Egg	440	27	980
Scrambled Eggs	140	10	290
Entrees			
"Big Mac"	560	32	950
Cheeseburger	310	14	750
"Chicken McNuggets" (6 pieces)	290	16	520
Barbeque Sauce	50	<1	340
Honey	45	0	0
Hot Mustard Sauce	70	4	250
Sweet and Sour Sauce	60	<1	190
"Filet-O-Fish"	440	26	1030
Hamburger	260	10	500
"McChicken"	490	29	780
"Mc D.L.T."	580	37	990
"Quarter Pounder"	410	21	660
"Quarter Pounder with Cheese"	520	29	1150
Side Dishes			
French Fries, Large	400	22	200
French Fries, Medium	320	17	150
French Fries, Small	220	12	110
Shakes and Desserts			
Apple Pie	260	15	240
Chocolaty Chip Cookies	330	16	280
Cone	140	4	70
McDonaldland Cookies	290	9	300
Shake, Chocolate	390	11	240
Shake, Strawberry	380	10	170
Shake, Vanilla	350	10	170
Soft Serve Sundae, Hot Caramel	340	9	160
Soft Serve Sundae, Hot Fudge	310	9	160
Soft Serve Sundae, Strawberry	280	7	80
Salads			
Chef Salad	230	13	490
Chicken Salad Oriental	140	3	230
Garden Salad	110	7	160
Side Salad	60	3	85
Bleu Cheese dressing (½ ounce)	70	7	150
Caesar dressing (½ ounce)	60	6	170
French dressing (½ ounce)	58	5	180
Lite Vinaigrette dressing (½ ounce)	15	<1	75
1000 Island dressing (½ ounce)	78	8	100
Oriental dressing (½ ounce)	24	<1	180

McDonald's (continued)

	Calories	FAT gm	Sodium gm
Peppercorn dressing (½ ounce)	80	9	85
Ranch dressing (½ ounce)	83	9	130
Red French Reduced Calorie dressing (½ ounce)	40	2	110
Beverages			
Coca-Cola Classic (16 ounces with ice)	190	*	20
Diet Coke (16 ounces with ice)	1	*	40
Grapefruit Juice (6 ounces)	80	0	0
Orange Drink (16 ounces with ice)	180	*	15
Orange Juice (6 ounces)	80	0	0
Sprite (16 ounces with ice)	190	*	20
2% Milk (8 ounces)	120	5	130

Pizza Hut

	Calories	FAT gm	Sodium gm
Pan Pizza			
Cheese, Medium, 2 slices	492	18	940
Pepperoni, Medium, 2 slices	540	22	1127
Supreme, Medium, 2 slices	589	30	1363
Super Supreme, Medium, 2 slices	563	26	1447
"Thin 'n Crispy" Pizza			
Cheese, Medium, 2 slices	398	17	867
Pepperoni, Medium, 2 slices	413	20	986
Supreme, Medium, 2 slices	459	22	1328
Hand-Tossed			
Cheese, Medium, 2 slices	518	20	1276
Pepperoni, Medium, 2 slices	500	23	1267
Supreme, Medium, 2 slices	540	26	1470
Super Supreme, Medium, 2 slices	556	25	1648
"Personal Pan Pizza"			
Pepperoni, whole pizza	675	29	1335
Supreme, whole pizza	647	28	1313

Ponderosa

	Calories	FAT gm	Sodium gm
Entrees			
Chicken Breast (5.5 oz.)[1]	98	2	400
Chicken Wings, 2 pieces	213	9	610
Chopped Steak (4 oz.)[1]	225	16	150
Chopped Steak (5.3 oz.)[1]	296	22	296
Fish, Baked			
Bake 'N Broil (5.2 oz.)	230	13	330
Baked Scrod (7 oz.)	120	1	80

[1] Pre-cooked weight. Nutritive value calculated on cooked weight.

* Indicates that information for this nutrient has not been analyzed or is not available.

Ponderosa (continued)

	Calories	FAT gm	Sodium gm
Fish, Broiled			
Halibut (6 oz.)	170	2	68
Roughy (5 oz.)	139	5	88
Salmon (6 oz.)	192	3	72
Swordfish (5.9 oz.)	271	9	*
Trout (5 oz.)	228	4	51
Fish, Fried (3.2 oz.)	190	9	170
Fish Nuggets, 1 piece	31	2	52
Hot Dog, (1.6)[1]	144	13	460
Kansas City Strip (5 oz.)[1]	138	6	850
New York Strip, Choice (10 oz.)[1]	314	14	1420
New York Strip, Choice (8 oz.)[1]	236	10	570
Porterhouse, Choice (16 oz.)[1]	640	31	1130
Ribeye, Choice (6 oz.)[1]	282	14	570
Sandwich steak (4 oz.)	408	11	850
Sirloin, Choice (7 oz.)[1]	241	11	570
Sirloin Tips, Choice (5 oz.)[1]	473	8	280
Steak Kabobs, Meat only (3 oz.)[1]	153	5	280
Teriyaki Steak (5 oz.)[1]	174	3	1420
T-Bone, Choice (10 oz.)[1]	444	18	850
Side Dishes			
Macaroni and Cheese, (1 oz.)	17	<1	80
Potatoes,			
Baked	145	<1	6
French Fried, (3 oz.)	120	4	39
Mashed, (4 oz.)	62	<1	191
Wedges, (3.5 oz.)	130	6	171
Rice Pilaf (4 oz.)	160	4	450
Rolls, Dinner	184	3	311
Rolls, Sourdough	110	1	230
Salad Dressings			
Blue Cheese, (1 oz.)	130	13	266
Creamy Italian, (1 oz.)	103	10	373
Parmesan Pepper, (1 oz.)	150	15	282
Ranch, (1 oz.)	147	15	298
Reduced Cal. Cucumber, (1 oz.)	69	6	316
Reduced Cal. Italian, (1 oz.)	31	3	371
Sour Cream, 1 Tbsp.	26	2	6
Sweet-n-Tangy	122	9	347
Thousand Island, (1 oz.)	113	10	405
Desserts			
Gelatin, Plain, (4 oz.)	152	3	70
Ice Milk, Chocolate (3.5 oz.)	71	0	73
Ice Milk, Vanilla (3.5 oz.)	150	3	58
Mousse, Chocolate (1 oz.)	80	4	18
Mousse, Strawberry (1 oz.)	74	5	17

[1] Pre-cooked weight. Nutritive value calculated on cooked weight.

* Indicates that information for this nutrient has not been analyzed or is not available.

Ponderosa (continued)

	Calories	FAT gm	Sodium gm
Toppings, Caramel (1 oz.)	100	<1	72
Chocolate (1 oz.)	89	<1	37
Strawberry (1 oz.)	71	<1	29
Whipped (1 oz.)	80	6	16
Beverages			
Caffeine Free Diet Coke, (6 oz.)	<1	0	8
Cherry Coke (6 oz.)	77	0	4
Coca-Cola (6 oz.)	72	0	7
Coffee (6 oz.)	2	0	26
Diet Coke (6 oz.)	<1	0	8
Diet Sprite (6 oz.)	2	0	4
Dr. Pepper (6 oz.)	72	0	14
Lemonade (6 oz.)	68	0	50
Milk, Chocolate (8 oz.)	208	8	149
White (8 oz.)	159	9	122
Mr. Pibb (6 oz.)	71	0	10
Orange (6 oz.)	82	0	0
Root Beer (6 oz.)	80	0	9
Sprite (6 oz.)	72	0	16

Rax

	Calories	FAT gm	Sodium gm
Entrees			
BBC (Beef, Bacon and Cheddar Sandwich)	720	49	1873
BBQ Sandwich	420	14	1343
Fish Sandwich	460	17	935
Ham and Swiss Sandwich	430	23	1737
Philly Beef and Cheese Sandwich	480	22	1346
Roast Beef Sandwich, Large	570	35	1169
Roast Beef Sandwich, Regular	320	11	969
Small Roast Beef Sandwich (Uncle Al)	260	14	562
Turkey Bacon Club	670	43	1878
BBQ Potato (2 oz. cheese)	730	24	1071
Cheese (3 oz.) and Bacon Potato	780	28	910
Cheese (3 oz.) and Broccoli Potato	760	26	489
Chili and Cheese (2 oz.) Potato	700	23	599
French Fries, Large (Salted)	390	20	104
French Fries, Regular (Salted)	260	13	69
Plain Potato	270	<1	70
Plain Potato with Margarine	370	11	170
Sour Topping Potato	400	11	149
Drive-thru Salads			
Chef Salad (without dressing)	230	14	1048
Garden Salad (without dressing)	160	11	362
Salad Bar			
Blue Cheese dressing (1 Tbsp.)	50	5	110
Cole Slaw (3.5 oz.)	70	4	187
French dressing (1 Tbsp.)	60	<4	140

Rax (continued)

	Calories	FAT gm	Sodium gm
Gelatin, Lime (½ cup)	90	<1	90
Gelatin, Strawberry (½ cup)	90	<1	90
Italian dressing (1 Tbsp.)	50	4	159
Lite Blue Cheese dressing (1 Tbsp.)	35	3	240
Lite French dressing (1 Tbsp.)	40	2	122
Lite Italian dressing (1 Tbsp.)	30	3	152
Lite Thousand Island dressing (1 Tbsp.)	40	3	143
Macaroni Salad (3.5 oz.)	160	7	216
Oil (1 Tbsp.)	130	14	<1
Pasta Salad (3.5 oz.)	80	1	322
Poppy Seed dressing (1 Tbsp.)	60	4	107
Potato Salad (1 cup)	260	17	127
Pudding, Butterscotch (3.5 oz.)	140	6	150
Pudding, Chocolate (3.5 oz.)	140	6	120
Pudding, Vanilla (3.5 oz.)	140	6	120
Ranch dressing (1 Tbsp.)	45	5	103
Mexican Bar			
Cheese Sauce, Regular (3.5 oz.)	420	17	365
Cheese Sauce, Nacho (3.5 oz.)	470	22	190
Refried Beans (3 oz.)	120	4	375
Sour Topping (3.5 oz.)	130	11	79
Spanish Rice (3.5 oz.)	90	<1	442
Spicy Meat Sauce (3.5 oz.)	80	4	751
Taco Sauce (3.5 oz.)	30	<1	806
Taco Shell	40	4	53
Tortilla	110	2	284
Tortilla Chips (1 oz.)	140	7	100
Pasta Bar			
Alfredo Sauce (3.5 oz.)	80	3	70
Chicken Noodle Soup (3.5 oz.)	40	<1	1040
Creme of Broccoli Soup (3.5 oz.)	50	2	219
Parmesan Cheese Substitute (1 oz.)	80	4	1000
Pasta Shells (3.5 oz.)	170	<4	2
Pasta/Vegetable Blend (3.5 oz.)	100	4	11
Rainbow Rotini (3.5 oz.)	180	4	9
Spaghetti (3.5 oz.)	140	4	1
Spaghetti Sauce (3.5 oz.)	80	<1	635
Spaghetti Sauce w/Meat (3.5 oz.)	150	8	419
Shakes and Desserts			
Chocolate Chip Cookies	130	6	65
Milkshake, Chocolate (without whip topping)	560	13	239
Milkshake, Strawberry (without whip topping)	560	13	226
Milkshake, Vanilla (without whip topping)	500	14	286
Whipped Topping, one dip	50	4	6

Taco Bell

	Calories	FAT gm	Sodium gm
Entrees			
Bean Burrito, Green Sauce	351	10	763

Taco Bell (continued)

	Calories	FAT gm	Sodium gm
Entrees			
Bean Burrito, Red Sauce	357	10	888
Beef Burrito, Green Sauce	398	17	926
Beef Burrito, Red Sauce	403	17	1051
Burrito Supreme, Green Sauce	407	18	796
Burrito Supreme, Red Sauce	413	18	921
Chicken Fajita	226	10	619
Cinnamon Crispas	259	15	127
Double Beef Burrito Supreme, Green Sauce	451	22	928
Double Beef Burrito, Red Sauce	457	22	1053
Enchirito, Green Sauce	381	54	993
Enchirito, Red Sauce	382	20	1243
Guacamole	34	2	113
Hot Taco Sauce, packet	3	<1	82
Jalapeno Pepper	20	<1	1370
Mexican Pizza	575	37	1031
Meximelt	266	15	689
Nachos	346	18	399
Nachos Bell Grande	648	35	997
Pico De Gallo	8	<1	88
Pintos and Cheese, Green Sauce	184	9	518
Pintos and Cheese, Red Sauce	190	9	642
Ranch Dressing	236	25	571
Salsa	18	<1	376
Soft Taco	228	12	516
Soft Taco Supreme	275	16	516
Sour Cream	46	4	*
Steak Fajita	234	11	485
Super Combo Taco	286	16	462
Taco	183	11	276
Taco Bellgrande	355	23	472
Taco Light	410	29	594
Taco Salad without Shell	502	31	1056
Taco Salad with Salsa	941	61	1662
Taco Salad with Salsa, without Shell	520	31	1431
Taco Sauce, Packet	2	<1	126
Tostado, Green Sauce	237	11	471
Tostado, Red Sauce	243	11	596

Wendy's

	Calories	FAT gm	Sodium gm
Breakfast Items			
Bacon, 2 strips	60	4	250
Breakfast Potatoes	360	22	745
Breakfast Sandwich	370	19	770

* Indicates that information for this nutrient has not been analyzed or is not available.

Wendy's (continued)

	Calories	FAT gm	Sodium gm
Buttermilk Biscuit	320	17	860
Danish, Cheese	430	21	500
Egg Fried, One	90	6	95
Eggs, Scrambled, 2 Eggs	190	12	160
French Toast, 2 slices	400	19	850
Omelet #1 - Ham & Cheese	290	21	570
Omelet #2 - Ham, Cheese & Mushrooms	250	17	405
Omelet #3 - Ham, Cheese, Onion & Green Pepper	280	19	485
Omelet #4 - Mushrooms, Onion & Green Pepper	210	15	200
Sausage, patty	200	18	405
White Toast with Margarine, 2 slices	250	9	410
Entrees			
Bacon Swiss Burger	710	44	1390
Big Classic	580	34	1015
Big Classic with Cheese	640	40	1310
Chicken Breast Filet	430	19	705
Chili	230	9	960
Crispy Chicken Nuggets - 6 pieces cooked in animal/vegetable oil	290	21	615
Kid's Meal Cheeseburger	320	15	805
Kid's Meal Hamburger (2 oz. patty)	260	9	510
Philly Swiss Burger	510	24	975
Single Cheeseburger with Everything	490	28	1100
Single Hamburger Patty (¼ lb.)	350	16	420
Single with Cheese	410	22	710
Single with Everything	430	22	805
Small Cheeseburger	320	15	805
Small Hamburger (2 oz. patty)	260	9	510
Taco Salad	660	37	1110
Take-Out Salads			
Chef Salad	180	9	140
Garden Salad	102	5	110
Side Dishes			
French Fries (cooked in animal/vegetable oil)	310	15	105
Bacon and Cheese Potato	570	30	1180
Broccoli and Cheese Potato	500	25	430
Cheese Potato	590	34	450
Chili and Cheese Potato	510	20	610
Plain Potato	250	2	60
Sour Cream and Chives Potato	460	24	230
Shakes and Desserts			
"Frosty" Dairy Dessert	400	14	220
"Garden Spot" Salad Bar			
California Cole slaw (2 oz.)	60	6	140
Deluxe Three Bean Salad (¼ cup)	60	<1	15
Old Fashion Corn Relish (¼ cup)	35	<1	205
Pasta Deli Salad (¼ cup)	35	<1	120
Red Bliss Potato Salad	110	9	265
Butterscotch Pudding (¼ cup)	90	4	85
Chocolate Pudding (¼ cup)	90	4	70

Wendy's (continued)

	Calories	FAT gm	Sodium gm
Blue Cheese dressing (1 Tbsp.)	80	9	90
Celery Seed dressing (1 Tbsp.)	70	6	65
Creamy Peppercorn (1 Tbsp.)	80	8	135
French dressing (1 Tbsp.)	70	6	190
Golden Italian dressing (1 Tbsp.)	50	4	260
"Hidden Valley" Ranch dressing (1 Tbsp.)	50	6	115
Italian Caesar dressing (1 Tbsp.)	70	8	125
Oil (Tbsp.)	120	14	0
Reduced Calorie Bacon and Tomato (1 Tbsp.)	45	4	190
Reduced Calorie Creamy Cucumber (1 Tbsp.)	50	5	140
Reduced Calorie Italian (1 Tbsp.)	25	2	180
Reduced Calorie Thousand Island (1 Tbsp.)	45	4	125
Sweet Red French Dressing (1 Tbsp.)	70	6	130
Thousand Island Dressing (1 Tbsp.)	70	7	105
Wine Vinegar (1 Tbsp.)	2	<1	5

21

CHEF EDWARD'S HINTS AND TIPS

K nowing and using the basic elements of food preparation are an important part of every meal. Meals are more than just eating food to keep our bodies going. Dining should be a pleasant experience. Meals do not need to be luxurious or fancy — a nicely done soup and salad luncheon can be a welcome break in a hectic day. Preparation and presentation are the keys to a memorable and enjoyable meal that you, your family and your friends will remember for a long time.

TEMPERATURE

This is the most basic element. Hot food should be served on hot plates. The food must be hot prior to plating and served immediately.

Cold food must be served on well-chilled plates and the food must be cold or kept on ice prior to serving.

REMEMBER: "Hot food served hot on hot plates."
"Cold food served cold on cold plates."

FLAVOR

All of the food on the plate is meant to be eaten. Therefore, all items must be well-seasoned and complement each other. Even though each individual food by itself might be well-prepared, if they do not complement each other, the meal will be undesirable.

COLOR

People eat with their eyes. In presenting food, you must keep in mind that multiple colors are much more appealing than foods that are similar in color. A plate with no contrasting colors looks dull, and gives the impression that it tastes dull too. Use naturally bright-colored foods and prepare them properly.

TEXTURE

The key to texture is variety. Your plate should include foods with many different textures. Not only for taste purposes, but also for eye appeal. Smooth, soft, crunchy, liquid, solid and firm textures should be used in a basic plate presentation. A well-balanced meal uses many textures to create a memorable experience.

SHAPES

Your presentation of food should utilize several different shapes. Use the natural shapes of food to highlight your presentation. Stay away from foods that have a similar shape. Also, wherever possible, add some height to your plate. This will create a completely different dimension.

GARNISH

This is the final touch to add before serving your meal. Use edible garnishes that complement your meal. Make them simple but creative. This will make a difference between having "dinner" or having a "dining experience."

MEASUREMENTS AND ABBREVIATIONS

tsp.	=	teaspoon
T	=	tablespoon
C	=	cup - 8 liquid ounces
oz.	=	ounce
gr.	=	gram
1 lb.	=	16 ounces
ea.	=	each
pt.	=	pint - 16 liquid ounces
qt.	=	quart - 32 liquid ounces
gal.	=	gallon - 128 liquid ounces

EQUIVALENTS

16 oz.	=	1 lb.
3 tsp.	=	1 T
16 T	=	1 C
2 C	=	1 pt.
2 pts.	=	1 qt.
4 qt.	=	1 gal.

THE BEST COOKING METHODS FOR LOW-FAT MEALS

POACHING: A method of gently cooking food completely covered in liquid (180-200 degrees).

For low-fat cooking, a defatted stock or bouillon is perfect. This should be seasoned with onions, celery and carrots and fresh herbs of your choice. Cook this liquid for 15-20 minutes to extract all of the flavors and strain. Use this liquid to poach your food items.

STEAMING: To cook food over a liquid that is boiling to create steam (212 degrees).

This is a terrific way to cook foods without adding fat. It preserves many nutrients and retains the natural flavor and color of many foods. There are many simple steaming units you can purchase for in-home use that are very easy to use.

BROILING: A transfer of heat through the air to brown and cook food.

This is an excellent method for cooking foods that have natural fat in them. Use a broiling rack to place food on to help eliminate excess fat. The major flavor given to food cooked with this method comes from the type of marinade you use on the food.

TIPS FOR LOW-FAT MEAL PREPARATION

1. Steam, poach or broil foods instead of sauteing, roasting or deep-fat frying.
2. If using any oils, think teaspoon instead of tablespoon.
3. Use skim milk instead of homogenized milk.
4. When cooking pastas, do not add oil to the water.
5. Use non-stick pans whenever possible to eliminate cooking with oils.
6. Use arrowroot or cornstarch for thickening instead of the animal or cooking fats used in rouxs.
7. Substitute fat-free food choices for high-fat foods.
8. Use fresh herbs in place of dried herbs if you can. They give a much better flavor.
9. Trim off all visual fat from any item that you are cooking.
10. Read all labels completely.
11. Choose meat labeled "very lean" or "extra lean."
12. Chill soups and stocks to make it easy to remove excess fat.
13. Use fat-free yogurts instead of low-fat yogurts.
14. Use flavored vinegars to season foods.
15. Purchase as many fresh products as possible.
16. Baste meats with defatted stocks instead of butter.
17. Make good use of stone-ground mustards, chutneys, lemon juice, garlic and onions.
18. Use a microwave to reheat leftover foods. This will eliminate adding fat to reheat.
19. If you use oils, try using infused oils. They add more flavor and you can get

away with using less.

20. Purchase low-fat or fat-free salad dressings. These make great dips as well as dressings for use on salads and pastas.

QUALITY POTS AND PANS - MY OTHER SECRET WEAPON

Aside from using herbs and spices to supercharge foods with flavor, the next most important item is good pots and pans. Today's non-stick cookware is a far cry from what was available even only a few years ago.

Today you can pick from more than 40 different lines of non-stick cookware. And non-stick cookware is really the only type to consider, especially for low-fat cooking.

Non-stick pans offer the best in the way of low-fat, or even no-fat, cooking. Foods don't stick, you can use very small amounts of oil if you want to and the pans clean up ever so nicely.

All non-stick pans offer quick clean-up, but that's about as far as their similarities go. Different manufacturers make pans that differ in durability, price and performance. Some don't cook as well as others, and some are less durable than their competitors.

So which should you buy? It really depends on your cooking habits and the money that you want to spend. Do you really enjoy cooking? Is it an important part of your life? Or do you just want pans that let you cook quick and easy meals for your family and friends?

Good sets that will serve you well can be had for as little as $100, or you can spend up to $400 for high-end professional pans. You'll most likely find what you need in any good department store cooking department or at a specialty cooking shops.

At a minimum, here's what you'll need:

1. Two saucepans with lids - pick the size you use most often (somewhere in the 3-5 quart range).

2. One saute pan, in the 10-12" size.

3. A one or two-burner griddle is very handy for vegetables, eggs, appetizers, small portions of meat and the ever-popular pancakes.

4. If you use them a lot, add specialty pieces such as an omelet pan or another saute pan.

TYPES OF PANS TO CONSIDER

Various types of pans are available. You can choose aluminum, cast or anodized aluminum, stainless steel and even glass.

I'd stay clear of the plain aluminum pans — they just aren't as durable. Coated cast or anodized aluminum is perhaps the very best heat conductor available. One warning: aluminum reacts with acidic foods like tomatoes, so be sure any aluminum pan is well coated with a non-aluminum, non-stick coating. Also make sure it covers the entire inside of the pan.

Stainless steel works well, but is not as good a heat conductor as aluminum. One way to solve this problem is to use stainless pans that have an aluminum or copper core to increase heat conductivity.

There are several non-stick coatings to choose from, and they all work well. Some companies spray on the coating, others dip the pan in the coating. Some manufacturers use one coat, others apply up to three coats of non-stick material. Obviously, the more the better.

Farberware sells nonstick pans made of stainless steel with an aluminum heat conductor on the bottom of the pan. These are good for browning and sauteing.

Millenium is popular with chefs, as is Excalibur and Castex. Excalibur is stainless steel, while Castex is anodized cast aluminum. Magnalite and Ultrex, both stainless steel with copper cores, are also popular.

Both Farberware and T-fal are popular for the home market due to their somewhat lower cost. T-fal's Resisteel, a stainless steel pan with a copper core, sells for about $170 for an eight-piece set.

Whichever brand you choose, they will all give you good service for years and the added benefit of low- or no-fat cooking and spotlessly quick cleanup!

SELECTED SOURCES OF
RELIABLE NUTRITION INFORMATION

American Dietetic Association
430 N. Michigan Ave.
Chicago, IL 60611

American Home Economics Association
Division of Public Affairs
2010 Massachusetts Ave. NW
Washington, DC 20036

American Institute of Baking
400 E. Ontario St.
Chicago, IL 60611

American Institute of Nutrition
9650 Rockville Pike
Bethesda, MD 20014

American Meat Institute
59 E. Van Buren St.
P.O. Box 3556
Washington, DC 20007

American Medical Association
Council on Foods and Nutrition
535 N. Dearborn St.
Chicago, IL 60610

American Public Health Association
1015 18th St. NW

Washington, DC 20036

American School Food Service
P.O. Box 10095
Denver, CO 80210

Children's Bureau
U.S. Department of Health, Education and Welfare
Washington, DC 20203

Food and Agriculture Organization (FAO) of the U.N.
c/o American Public Health Association
1740 Broadway
New York, NY 10019

Food and Drug Administration (FDA)
Parkland Building
5600 Fishers Lane
Rockville, MD 20852

Food and Nutrition Board
National Academy of Sciences
2101 Constitution Ave.
Washington, DC 20418

National Dietary Council
6300 N. River Rd.
Rosemont, IL 60018

National Foundation - March of Dimes
Health Information Department
P.O. Box 2000
White Plains, NY 10602

National Livestock and Meat Board
444 N. Michigan Ave.
Chicago, IL 60611

National Nutrition Consortium
24 Third St. NE Suite 200
Washington, DC 20002

Nutrition Foundation, Inc.
888 17th St. NW
Washington, DC 20016

Nutrition Information and Resource Center
Benedict House
Pennsylvania State University
University Park, PA 16802

Nutrition Today Society
101 Ridgly Ave.
P.O. Box 773
Annapolis, MD 21404

Society for Nutrition Education
1736 Franklin St.
Oakland, CA 94612

Superintendent of Documents
U.S. Government Printing Office
Washington, DC 20402

U.S. Department of Agriculture
Cooperative Extension Service
Home Economics
Washington, DC 20250

Nutrition Program Consumer and Food Economics Division
Agricultural Research Service
Hyattsville, MD 20782

Office of Communications
Washington, DC 20250

School Lunch Program
Information Division
Food and Nutrition Service
Washington, DC 20250

World Health Organization (WHO)
Distribution and Sales Service
1211 Geneva 27, Switzerland

Your local Cooperative Extension Service may also have free information available to give to you.

A FIRST-EVER FROM BIOTECH:

THE GREEN, YELLOW AND RED ZONE FOOD TABLE, RANKING FOODS BY FAT AND CALORIES

Thiis exclusive food chart represents a comparison of fat grams and calories based on a proprietary formula developed by Biotech researchers in our test kitchen.

This is the first ranking of foods by fat grams and calories that uses a common unit of measure for all the foods. All food values listed are for an 8 ounce serving. If you eat more or less than this amount, use the 8 ounce value and simply multiply or divide according to your individual serving size.

Use this table as a guide for choosing foods to eat. The first table is in ascending order by fat grams. The second table is an alphabetical listing of foods, with the Green-Yellow-Red Zone noted for each individual food.

Green Zone foods should form the basis for most of your daily food intake. They are low in both fat and calories.

Yellow Zone foods should be eaten in moderation. The caloric content of Yellow Zone foods is still rather low, but in most cases the fat grams are noticeably higher than Green Zone foods.

Red Zone foods should be eaten very sparingly. For these foods, the fat grams and calories are at much higher levels when compared to Green or Yellow Zone foods. We suggest using these foods only for those special occasions, such as a special dinner at your favorite restaurant on your birthday or anniversary, and family gatherings at home on holidays.

Food	Per 8 ozs. Fat grams	Calories
Soft drink, 7-Up, diet	0.0	0
Soft drink, club soda	0.0	0
Spinach, cooked	0.0	0
Spinach, fresh	0.0	1
Celery, fresh	0.0	2
Soft drink, Fresca	0.0	4
Endive	0.0	4
Cabbage, cooked	0.0	4
Potatoes, peeled, grated	0.0	4
Coffee, regular	0.0	4
Cabbage, fresh, grated	0.0	5
Alfalfa sprouts	0.0	5
Bamboo shoots, LaChoy	0.0	6
Gravy, brown mix	0.0	8
Chinese cabbage	0.0	10
Coffee, instant	0.0	11
Pear, Balsam, raw	0.0	15
Chicory	0.0	15
Chives	0.0	16
Vinegar, Whitehouse apple cider	0.0	16
Radish, fresh	0.0	17
Celery, diced, cooked	0.0	20
Mustard greens, fresh, boiled	0.0	22
Broccoli, fresh	0.0	24
Collards	0.0	24
Tomato, fresh	0.0	26
Green beans, snapped, canned	0.0	26
Dandelion greens, raw, chopped	0.0	26
Eggplant, fresh, boiled	0.0	26
Zucchini squash, fresh	0.0	28
Zucchini squash, cooked	0.0	28
Mushrooms, fresh	0.0	29
Iceberg lettuce, shredded	0.0	30
Pumpkin, raw, cubed	0.0	30
Cauliflower, cooked	0.0	30
Mung beans, sprouted seeds, raw	0.0	32
Cucumber	0.0	32
Pickles, zesty dill spears	0.0	32
Pokeberry shoots, fresh, cooked	0.0	32
Vinegar, Regina, red wine	0.0	32
Dandelion greens, cooked	0.0	34
Sharps non-alcoholic beer	0.0	34

EAT GREEN ZONE FOODS MOST OFTEN

| | Per 8 ozs. | |
Food	Fat grams	Calories
Cauliflower, fresh	0.0	38
Grapefruit, fresh	0.0	38
Kohlrabi, raw	0.0	38
Green peppers, fresh	0.0	38
Brussels sprouts, cooked	0.0	40
Brussels sprouts, fresh	0.0	40
Broccoli, cooked	0.0	44
Yellow beans	0.0	44
Strawberries, fresh	0.0	45
Dock, cooked	0.0	45
Carrots, fresh, shredded	0.0	48
Turnip greens, cooked	0.0	48
Onions, fresh green	0.0	48
Onions, fresh white	0.0	50
Rutabaga, raw	0.0	50
Cardoon	0.0	51
Watermelon	0.0	52
Cranberries, fresh	0.0	54
Mandarin orange-flavored drink, Koala	0.0	55
Sauerkraut, canned	0.0	56
Asparagus, fresh	0.0	60
Honeydew, fresh, cubed	0.0	60
Raspberries, red, fresh	0.0	60
Pimientos	0.0	60
Asparagus, cooked	0.0	60
Boysenberries, fresh	0.0	62
Celeriac root (wild celery)	0.0	62
Leeks, raw	0.0	64
Ale, brown, bottled	0.0	66
Lime juice	0.0	66
Bok Choy	0.0	68
Okra, fresh cooked	0.0	68
Peas, snow	0.0	68
Pumpkin, canned	0.0	70
Pomelo, raw	0.0	71
Currants, raw	0.0	72
Beer, Budweiser lite	0.0	73
Grapes, fresh	0.0	74
Figs, fresh	0.0	74
Blackberries, fresh	0.0	74
Shell beans	0.0	74
Pineapple, fresh	0.0	76
Fruit salad, water packed	0.0	80

EAT GREEN ZONE FOODS MOST OFTEN

Food	Per 8 ozs. Fat grams	Calories
Casaba melon	0.0	80
Cherries, fresh sweet	0.0	80
Juice, body quencher, All Sports	0.0	80
Mixed vegetables, Libby's	0.0	80
Ginger beer	0.0	80
Papaya, fresh pulp	0.0	80
Fruit cocktail, mixed	0.0	80
Apple, fresh	0.0	81
Blueberries, fresh	0.0	82
Tonic water	0.0	85
Loganberries	0.0	90
Yogurt, Weight Watchers, all flavors	0.0	90
Collins mix, Schweppes	0.0	93
Coca Cola	0.0	93
Orange, fresh	0.0	96
Baking powder	0.0	96
Paprika seasoning	0.0	96
Salsa, Ortega medium green chili	0.0	96
Sugar Twin, white and brown	0.0	96
Beer, regular	0.0	96
Pears, fresh	0.0	97
Popped corncakes, cheddar	0.0	100
Eggbeaters egg substitute	0.0	100
Lemon sour mix, Schweppes	0.0	100
Parsnips, raw	0.0	100
Pineapple juice, Bluebird, 100% pure juice	0.0	100
Caramel corn cakes	0.0	100
Applesauce, unsweetened	0.0	104
Yogurt, blueberry, non-fat lite, Dannon	0.0	109
Yambean, boiled	0.0	110
Orange juice, Minutemaid	0.0	110
Mixed fruit, water packed	0.0	112
Orange drink, powder, prepared with water	0.0	115
Cider, 6.9% alcohol	0.0	116
Ice pop, lime, Hershey's	0.0	120
Soy sauce	0.0	120
Cream soda	0.0	120
Jello-O, regular	0.0	122
Ketchup, low salt, Heinz	0.0	128
Basil seasoning	0.0	144
Basil, French's	0.0	144
Croutons, Kellogg's	0.0	144

Food	Per 8 ozs.	
	Fat grams	Calories
Cranapple juice, Oceanspray	0.0	160
Butter beans	0.0	160
Figs, canned in light syrup	0.0	174
Kidney beans, canned	0.0	180
Cantaloupe, fresh	0.0	180
Peaches, Del Monte, heavy syrup	0.0	180
Champagne	0.0	180
Blackeyed peas, cooked	0.0	180
Baby lima beans	0.0	186
Broad beans	0.0	186
Mung beans, boiled	0.0	190
Bananas, fresh, whole	0.0	190
Garlic powder seasoning	0.0	192
Concord grape jelly, S&W	0.0	192
Orange marmalade, S&W	0.0	192
Strawberry jam, S&W	0.0	192
Cannellini beans	0.0	192
Applesauce, sweetened	0.0	194
Chocolate mocha, Ultra Slim Fast, skim milk	0.0	200
Yardlong beans	0.0	204
Corn, canned	0.0	206
Lemon ice, Ben & Jerry's	0.0	208
Kidney beans	0.0	218
Potato, plain baked	0.0	218
Lobster, northern, cooked	0.0	220
Mixed vegetables, canned, Hanover	0.0	220
Raspberry sorbet, Dole	0.0	220
Red beans, cooked	0.0	224
Cow peas, frozen, cooked	0.0	224
Black beans	0.0	228
Lentils	0.0	232
Baking soda	0.0	240
Rice Chex cereal, Ralston	0.0	240
Bread & butter pickles, Vlasic	0.0	240
Relish, sweet, Vlasic	0.0	240
Bay leaf seasoning	0.0	240
Bay leaf	0.0	240
Daiquiri (2)	0.0	248
Prunes, canned, heavy syrup	0.0	248
Beans, pink, boiled	0.0	248
Dressing, fat-free, whipped, Weight Watchers	0.0	258
Raspberries, red, frozen	0.0	258
Refried beans	0.0	260

EAT GREEN ZONE FOODS MOST OFTEN

Food	Fat grams	Calories
Ranch, free salad dressing, Kraft	0.0	260
Poi	0.0	268
Plums, whole, canned	0.0	270
Cassava root, raw	0.0	274
Sherry	0.0	280
Garlic powder	0.0	288
Allspice	0.0	288
Ketchup, Heinz	0.0	288
Ginger seasoning	0.0	288
Wine, dessert, dry 18.8% alcohol	0.0	299
Miracle Whip, fat-free	0.0	320
Pretzels, Shearer's	0.0	320
Waffles, Special K	0.0	320
Wine, sweet	0.0	356
Wine, dessert sweet, 18.8% alcohol	0.0	363
Cream of tartar	0.0	368
Pancake/waffle syrup, lite, Aunt Jemima	0.0	400
Cornmeal, white or yellow	0.0	400
Cracker meal	0.0	400
Syrup, Weight Watchers	0.0	400
Pinto beans, frozen, cooked	0.0	405
Currants, dried	0.0	408
Flour, arrowroot	0.0	464
Cinnamon, ground	0.0	480
Flour, bread	0.0	495
Lemon curd	0.0	528
Gin, rum, vodka, 80 proof	0.0	549
Applebutter, Smucker's	0.0	560
Marshmallows, Kraft	0.0	560
Gin, rum, vodka, 90 proof	0.0	624
Triple Sec	0.0	632
Molasses, blackstrap	0.0	640
Chutney, apple	0.0	656
Sloe gin	0.0	661
Peppermint Schnapps, liqueur	0.0	661
Brandy, fruit flavor	0.0	688
Gin, rum, vodka, 100 proof	0.0	698
Breading frying mix	0.0	720
Sugar, white, granulated	0.0	770
Honey	0.0	773
Anisette, liqueur	0.0	789
Onion ring mix	0.0	800
Quaker puffed wheat (8 cups)	0.0	800

EAT GREEN ZONE FOODS MOST OFTEN

| | Per 8 ozs. | |
Food	Fat grams	Calories
Sugar, brown, packed	0.0	821
Candy corn	0.0	824
Jelly, concord grape, Welch's	0.0	840
Jam, Smucker's, all flavors	0.0	864
Pancake and waffle syrup, Aunt Jemima	0.0	880
Drambuie liqueur	0.0	880
Pancake and waffle syrup, Golden Griddle	0.0	885
Dates, dried	0.0	912
Karo syrup, lite corn	0.0	928
Karo syrup	0.0	960
Molasses, Brer Rabbit, black and white	0.0	960
Creme de menthe liqueur	0.0	992
Tea, cinnamon stick, regular, Bigelow	Tr.	1
Tea, orange, spice, herbal, Bigelow	Tr.	1
Watercress, chopped	Tr.	2
Tea, amaretto, Celestial regular tea	Tr.	3
Tea, cinnamon, apple spice, Celestial	Tr.	3
Sesbania flowers	Tr.	5
Purslane, raw	Tr.	7
Cabbage, swamp, raw, chopped	Tr.	11
Purslane, cooked	Tr.	21
Sesbania flowers, cooked	Tr.	23
Turnip greens, raw, frozen	Tr.	34
Turnip greens, raw	Tr.	36
Melon balls, frozen	Tr.	55
Java plum	Tr.	82
Kellogg's Special K cereal	Tr.	83
Tangerine, fresh	Tr.	86
Kellogg's Corn Flakes cereal	Tr.	88
Clams, chopped, canned	Tr.	110
Passion fruit juice	Tr.	126
Jackfruit	Tr.	160
Sweet potato, canned in syrup	Tr.	183
Ultra Slim Fast, French vanilla, skim milk	Tr.	190
Ultra Slim Fast, French vanilla, prepared	Tr.	220
Tequila Sunrise	0.1	252
Pasta shell, dried, Mueller's	0.1	840
Tomato juice	0.2	41
Artichoke, plain	0.2	53
V-8 Juice	0.2	53
Apple juice, Mott's	0.2	117
Milk, skim	0.4	86
Orange juice, fresh squeezed	0.4	112

EAT GREEN ZONE FOODS MOST OFTEN

| | Per 8 ozs. | |
Food	Fat grams	Calories
Yogurt, non-fat	0.4	127
Angelfood cake	0.4	166
Enchilada, chicken, frozen, Banquet	0.4	247
Chestnuts, roasted	0.4	560
Pitanga	0.6	57
Soup, clam chowder, Manhattan	0.6	66
Salsa, Chi Chi's mild	0.6	72
Mango, fruit, diced	0.6	109
Strawberry sorbet	0.6	142
Barley, cooked	0.6	193
Rice, white, cooked	0.6	264
Pierogi, onion	0.6	480
Apple fruit snack, Weight Watcher's	0.6	800
Jelly beans	0.6	832
Log Cabin syrup, buttered	0.6	848
Cloves, seasoning	0.7	110
Gooseberries, raw	0.8	67
Elderberries, raw	0.8	105
Dates, chopped	0.8	489
Watercress, chopped	0.9	4
Swiss chard, fresh	0.9	6
Postum, instant, prepared	0.9	14
Cabbage, swamp, cooked	0.9	16
Chinese vegetables, LaChoy	0.9	20
Zucchini squash, raw sliced	0.9	28
Zucchini squash, Italian style	0.9	28
Swiss chard, cooked	0.9	36
Kale	0.9	40
Tomatillo, fresh	0.9	42
Tree fern, chopped, cooked	0.9	56
Mulberries	0.9	61
Chinese water chestnuts	0.9	70
Rose apple, fresh	0.9	73
Ground cherries, fresh	0.9	74
Bloody Mary mix, with Tabasco	0.9	75
Mixed vegetables, homemade	0.9	78
Burdock root, raw	0.9	85
Guava sauce	0.9	86
Sunkist funfruit	0.9	89
Plums, fresh sliced	0.9	91
Peas and carrots, homemade	0.9	96
Sage	0.9	96
Burdock root, cooked	0.9	110

EAT GREEN ZONE FOODS MOST OFTEN

| | Per 8 ozs. | |
Food	Fat grams	Calories
Taro, raw sliced	0.9	112
Feijoa, fresh	0.9	114
Rhubarb, frozen	0.9	120
Yam, cubed, cooked	0.9	158
Jujube, raw	0.9	184
Taro, cooked	0.9	188
Rosemary, dried	0.9	192
Macaroni, cooked	0.9	197
Ultra Slim chocolate pudding, prepared	0.9	200
Cranberry beans	0.9	216
Chocolate Instant Breakfast with skim milk	0.9	220
French beans, dried	0.9	228
Pepper	0.9	240
Ginkgo nuts, canned	0.9	256
Navy beans, boiled	0.9	258
Tamarind, fresh, cut up	0.9	287
Curry seasoning	0.9	288
Poultry seasoning	0.9	288
Pumpkin pie spice	0.9	288
Pickles, sweet gerkin	0.9	320
Sweet potato, fresh, mashed	0.9	344
Yams, candied, canned	0.9	360
Cumin seasoning	0.9	384
Flour, cake	0.9	395
Yeast, brewer's dried	0.9	400
Ginkgo nuts, raw	0.9	416
Coffeemate powder	0.9	480
Log Cabin syrup, lite	0.9	488
Molasses, Grandma's Green or Gold label	0.9	1120
Rhubarb	1.0	60
Shrimp creole dinner, Amour	1.0	185
Bran, Miller's processed	1.0	186
Salt seasoning	1.0	192
White beans	1.0	254
Prunes, dried	1.0	380
Zucchini squash, cooked	1.3	20
Kelp, raw	1.3	49
Chow mein, beef, LaChoy	1.3	93
Bread crumbs, soft	1.3	122
Salsa, chunky mild, Rosarita	1.3	133
Garlic salt	1.3	144
Cocoa, Swiss Miss prepared with milk	1.3	147
Borage, raw	2.0	18

| | Per 8 ozs. | |
Food	Fat grams	Calories

MOST OFTEN

Borage, cooked	2.0	50
Vegetable soup, Campbell's condensed	2.0	90
Feijoa puree	2.0	119
Quaker oatmeal, cooked	2.0	145
Adzuki beans, boiled	2.0	149
Beans, Great Northern, canned	2.0	180
Pinto beans, Green Giant, canned	2.0	180
Corn pudding, homemade	2.0	194
Succotash, homemade	2.0	204
Succotash, S&W country style	2.0	204
Egg noodles, cooked	2.0	208
Pollack, raw	2.0	208
Vega burger, Loma Linda	2.0	220
Yogurt, frozen, TCBY	2.0	220
Cod, canned	2.0	237
Corn dogs, Loma Linda	2.0	251
Sherbet, lime	2.0	260
Chinese noodles, dried	2.0	585
Pink beans, raw	2.0	720
Cottage cheese, 1% fat	2.2	162
Chicken noodle soup, Campbell's	2.4	72
Shrimp, steamed	2.4	224
Jujube, dried	2.4	640
Clam chowder, New England	2.5	87
Chocolate milk, 1% fat	2.5	102
Milk, 1%	2.5	158
Stuffing, Brownberry	2.5	200
Cod, frozen	2.5	293
Coconut, angel flake	2.6	110
Breadsticks, traditional, whole wheat	2.6	160
Frogs' legs, raw	2.6	168
Scallops	2.6	185
Beef tenderloin, raw	2.6	187
Crab, raw	2.6	189
Sole, raw	2.6	205
Beef flank steak, lean, raw	2.6	213
Beef top round, raw	2.6	213
Alaskan crab, canned	2.6	219
Yogurt, low-fat, fruit	2.6	225
Perch, cooked	2.6	264
Seaweed, dried, Agar	2.6	693
Ameranth, box mix	2.8	149
Moth beans, cooked	3.0	70

EAT IN MODERATION

| | Per 8 ozs. | |
Food	Fat grams	Calories
Yogurt, all flavors, Cabot	3.0	110
Baked beans	3.0	120
Chinese fried rice, homemade	3.0	206
Sugar apple, fresh, cut up	3.0	236
Bluefish, raw	3.0	240
Baked beans, Campbell's	3.0	240
Pina colada	3.0	349
Popcorn, hot-air popped	3.0	369
Pizza, French bread and cheese, Healthy Choice	3.0	408
Cole slaw	3.2	82
Chicken noodles dinner, Banquet	3.2	136
Chocolate, Slender	3.2	176
Yogurt, frozen, all flavors, Bressler's	3.2	216
Yogurt, frozen, all flavors, Bressler's gourmet	3.2	232
Beef pepper steak, Healthy Choice	3.4	211
Roll, submarine	3.4	263
Sole, cooked	3.4	264
Flounder, cooked	3.4	266
Buttermilk	3.5	125
Peas, pigeon, fresh cooked	3.5	125
Flatfish, cooked	3.5	266
Beans, French, raw	4.0	52
Tomato soup, Campbell's condensed	4.0	140
Sirloin strip style dinner, Jaclyn's	4.0	172
Dynatrim, chocolate, prepared with 1% milk	4.0	220
Chick peas	4.0	268
Orange sherbet	4.0	270
Ritz crackers	4.0	476
Bread, white, regular (8 slices)	4.0	480
English muffins, sourdough	4.0	480
Yogurt, apple, Yoplait original	4.0	480
Lasagna	4.0	840
Macaroni	4.0	840
Spaghetti	4.0	840
Vermicelli	4.0	840
Beef stroganoff lite dinner, Armour	4.2	178
Enchilada, beef, frozen, Weight Watchers	4.4	167
Cottage cheese, 2% fat	4.4	204
Tofu, Mori-Nu extra firm	4.6	137
Chicken, Le Menu, Empress, lite	4.8	203
Evaporated milk, Carnation low-fat	4.8	216
Lotus seed	4.8	752
Crab, Dungeness canned	4.9	199

Food	Per 8 ozs.	
	Fat grams	Calories
Chicken a la King dinner, Armour	4.9	200
Milk, Vitamite, Deihl	5.0	100
Chocolate milk, homemade, 2% milk	5.0	179
Chocolate milk, commercial, 2% fat	5.0	179
Milk, 2%	5.0	180
Nestle's Quik chocolate with 2% milk	5.0	210
Gizzards, chicken, simmered	5.0	222
Pike, northern, cooked	5.0	261
Pigs' feet	5.0	395
Beef, chuck roast, lean, raw	5.3	213
Beef, eye of the round, raw	5.3	213
Beef, rib eye, raw	5.3	240
Pierogi, cheese	5.3	583
Gravy, beef, canned	5.6	120
Tofu, Mori-Nu soft	6.0	122
Tofu, Mori-Nu firm	6.0	137
Strawberry ice cream, Bryers	6.0	220
Turkey gizzards, simmered	6.0	236
Pasta salad, Lite Italian, with dressing, Kraft	6.0	260
Evaporated milk, regular	6.0	338
Pheasant	6.4	235
Chocolate milkshake	6.4	282
Enchilada, cheese, frozen, Banquet	6.5	249
Lamb stew, take-out	6.7	165
Hot cocoa mix, Nestle's, 2% milk	6.7	280
Beef noodles and gravy, Banquet	6.9	206
Acerola juice	7.0	51
Mushrooms, sauteed with 1 Tbls. margarine	7.0	60
Carob	7.0	140
Lamb stew, homemade	7.0	165
Milkshake, vanilla	7.1	265
Chicken, light meat, skinless, roasted	7.2	357
Yogurt, plain, regular	7.4	138
Bran, Quaker Oat	7.6	330
Kidney, simmered	7.7	325
Asparagus soup with milk	7.9	161
Milk, imitation	8.0	150
Homemade chocolate milk	8.0	208
Chocolate milk, Land o' Lakes	8.0	210
Chicken dumpling dinner, Banquet	8.0	216
Cool Whip cream topping	8.0	224
Beef sirloin tip, raw	8.0	240
Yogurt, blueberry, Yoplait original	8.0	240

EAT IN MODERATION

Food	Per 8 ozs.	
	Fat grams	Calories
Oyster crackers	8.0	240
Quail breast, no skin	8.0	276
Chocolate Instant Breakfast with whole milk	8.0	280
Tapioca	8.0	290
Custard, flan, Spanish style with milk	8.0	296
Chocolate pudding, regular	8.0	300
Rice pudding	8.0	310
Breadsticks, Stella Dora	8.0	320
Eggnog, Carnation lite	8.0	320
Tuna, packed in water	8.0	360
Shoestring potatoes, Ore Ida	8.0	400
Egg Pro, regular	8.0	440
White bread, Schwebel's (6 slices)	8.0	560
Breadsticks, Italian soft	8.0	640
Fettuccine, prepared	8.0	693
Noodles, egg/spinach	8.0	836
Ravioli with beef	8.0	900
Milk, whole, 3.3% fat	8.1	14
Swedish meatballs with sauce, Dining Delight	8.8	249
Chocolate milk, Hershey's whole milk	9.0	210
Chocolate malted milk	9.0	229
Nestle's ready-to-drink Quik	9.0	230
Swordfish, raw	9.0	275
Beef, New York strip	9.1	304
Pasta salad with vegetables	9.1	320
Ham steak dinner, Armour	9.5	255
Goose liver	9.6	303
Yogurt, Ben & Jerry's frozen cherry	9.6	320
Spaghetti sauce, Ragu, meatless	10.0	180
Strawberry ice cream	10.0	232
Winged beans, cooked	10.0	252
Spaghetti sauce, Prego	10.0	260
Pudding, Jell-O instant butterscotch	10.0	336
Rigatoni, prepared	10.4	533
Saltine crackers (64)	10.6	132
Beef liver	10.6	365
Pork liver	10.6	376
French toast, Aunt Jemima	10.6	442
Nestle's Quik chocolate powder	10.6	960
Beans and Franks dinner, Banquet	11.2	280
Bluefin fish, fresh	11.2	325
Turkey giblets	11.2	389
Macaroni salad, take out	11.4	366

Food	Per 8 ozs.	
	Fat grams	Calories
Turkey pastrami, thin sliced	11.6	276
Chocolate mocha pie, Weight Watchers	11.6	524
Chicken and dumplings, Swanson frozen	11.7	235
Glazed chicken dinner, Armour	11.9	238
Tofu, regular	12.0	176
Buttermilk biscuits	12.0	240
Tempeh	12.0	320
Yellowtail	12.0	330
Pudding, Swiss Miss chocolate prepared	12.0	60
Nutra shake, chocolate	12.0	400
Handy Pocket cheese sauce/ham, Weight Watchers	12.0	400
Wheat germ, plain, toasted	12.0	431
Egg noodles	12.0	880
Fettuccine	12.0	880
Egg noodles, Creamette	12.0	884
Mexican style dinner, Banquet	12.4	298
Trout	12.5	312
Carp, fresh	12.8	288
Giblets, capon	12.8	381
Beef heart, simmered	12.8	397
Tamales, beef, frozen, Banquet	13.0	305
Flavor Tree fruit bears	13.0	891
Chicken gravy, canned	13.6	192
French toast, home recipe	14.0	310
Croissant, Pepperidge Farm	14.0	340
Pizza, cheese, Kid Cuisine	14.0	444
Vanilla ice cream, regular	14.4	268
Chocolate ice cream	14.4	310
Jack mackerel, canned, drained	14.4	354
Salmon	14.4	833
Enchilada frozen beef dinner, Patio	14.5	314
Baked custard, homemade	14.6	305
Beef stew, Chef Boyardee	14.9	251
Canadian bacon	15.8	356
Hershey's Orange Blossom ice cream bar	16.0	293
Tamales with sauce, Van Camps	16.0	293
Vanilla ice cream, Bryers	16.0	300
Chocolate ice cream, Bryers	16.0	320
Italian pasta salad, take-home	16.0	320
Turkey, ground, fried	16.0	320
Turkey, ground, fresh	16.0	320
Tofu, Spring Creek barbecue baked	16.0	352
Nutri Balance frozen chocolate pudding	16.0	450

EAT IN MODERATION

EAT VERY RARELY

| | Per 8 ozs. | |
Food	Fat grams	Calories
Rykrisp	16.0	540
Miso paste	16.0	570
Honey butter, Downey's original	16.0	800
Breadsticks, Oro Wheat cheese	16.0	880
Graham crackers (16 crackers)	16.0	960
Hot roll mix, Pillsbury	16.0	960
Shake and Bake, fish	16.0	1184
Shake and Bake, pork	16.0	1280
Chicken, dark meat, no skin, roasted	16.3	424
Oysters, eastern, canned	16.8	157
Phyllo dough	17.0	815
Chicken and noodles, home recipe	18.0	365
Beef chili beans, Chef Boyardee	18.1	352
Tuna salad, take-out	19.0	383
Leg o' lamb, lean, roasted	19.0	432
Waffles, buttermilk, frozen, Aunt Jemima	19.2	573
Natto	19.4	374
Evaporated milk, regular	20.0	338
Burrito, crisp fried, Van de Camp	20.0	487
Rolls, home recipe	20.0	800
Pound cake	20.1	351
Herring, raw	20.2	357
Biscuits, mixed with milk	20.8	728
Zucchini squash, breaded, Ore Ida	21.0	400
Hummus, homemade	21.0	420
Corn muffins, Dromedary	21.3	640
Waffles, frozen, Multi-Grain, Weight Watchers	21.3	640
Salisbury steak with gravy, Banquet	21.7	297
Beef, extra lean ground	22.0	404
Franks, big meatless, Loma Linda	22.2	444
Hershey's Neo Wave ice cream bar	22.4	512
Tuna melt, Chefwich	22.4	576
Lamb curry, homemade	23.0	460
Brazil nuts	23.2	230
Vanilla ice cream, rich	23.6	350
Spaghetti sauce, Ragu thick and zesty	23.8	222
Vanilla wafers, Murray	24.0	64
Mayonnaise, home recipe	24.0	100
Olives, ripe	24.0	240
Franks, turkey links	24.0	360
Turkey pot pie, Swanson's	24.0	434
Croissant, home recipe	24.0	470
Olive loaf, Loma Linda	24.0	476

Food	Per 8 ozs. Fat grams	Calories
Cheese, Weight Watcher's sharp cheddar	24.0	560
Mozzarella cheese substitute	24.0	560
Lemon Fi-Bar	24.0	720
Bacon bits, Betty Crocker	24.0	600
Macaroni and cheese, take out	24.1	406
Ham, picnic	24.2	312
Meatless swiss steak with gravy, Loma Linda	24.6	431
Waffles, mix prepared with egg and milk	24.6	631
Eggs, raw, medium	24.9	369
Chicken pot pie, Swanson's	25.1	434
Pigs' ears	25.9	396
Chocolate ice cream, Baskin Robbins	26.0	528
Cherry pie, Sara Lee homestyle	26.0	540
Sardines	26.2	457
Apple pie, Banquet	26.6	606
Tamales, Wolf brand	27.0	350
Blueberry pie, Banquet	27.0	655
Chicken ravioli, prepared	27.0	693
Muffins, blueberry, home recipe	27.0	720
Omelette, Chefwich cheese	27.2	608
Vanilla ice cream, Baskin Robbins	28.0	480
Beef brains, simmered	28.2	363
Goose, skinless	28.8	544
Hershey's Ice cream sandwich (3)	28.8	672
Ham, country cured	29.0	461
Waffles, Eggo frozen buttermilk	29.0	756
Waffles, Eggo frozen homestyle	29.0	756
Avocado, California, fresh	29.8	306
Cornbread, prepared from mix	30.0	987
Three Musketeers, chocolate bar	30.5	990
Pistachio nuts, dry roasted	30.8	368
Nutri Grain apple breakfast bar	30.8	923
Half and Half, Land o' Lakes	32.0	320
Avocado guacomole dip, Kraft	32.0	400
Nacho cheese dip, Kraft	32.0	440
French onion dip, Hormel	32.0	440
Homestyle pasta salad with dressing, Kraft	32.0	480
Vegetable with chicken pot pie, Morton's	32.0	480
Bacon bits, Hormel	32.0	480
Chicken cacciatore, take-out	32.0	525
Ground round	32.0	573
Sweetbreads, veal, braised	32.0	581
Bran muffins, homemade	32.0	667

WATCH OUT — EAT VERY RARELY

Food	Per 8 ozs.	
	Fat grams	Calories
Bacon bits, Oscar Mayer	32.0	672
Corn muffins	32.0	773
Scone, plain	32.0	827
Hot fudge topping, Kraft	32.0	1120
Cheese curls, Weight Watcher's	32.0	1120
Shake and Bake, chicken	32.0	1200
Pate, chicken liver, canned	32.0	1904
Scrambled eggs, Kid Cuisine	33.1	527
Popcorn with oil and salt (17 cups)	34.0	697
Veal parmigiana	34.2	531
Pork chop, lean with fat	34.3	619
Pepperoni pizza, Celeste	34.3	640
Lamb sweetbreads, braised	34.6	534
Pizza, Celeste supreme	34.6	613
Hershey's choc. eclair crunch ice cream bar (2 1/2)	34.6	640
Polish kielbasa, Mr. Turkey	35.0	472
Nibbles, cherry and chocolate	35.0	1028
Beef pot pie, Morton's	35.4	494
Ham croquettes, home recipe	36.0	560
Fondu, take-out	36.0	606
Lobster Newburg	37.0	464
Italian sausage roll, frozen, Ovenstuffs	37.0	857
Quail breast, with skin	37.1	442
Beef chuck arm roast, braised	37.8	635
French vanilla ice cream, Baskin Robbins	38.0	580
Apple pie, Sara Lee homestyle	38.0	653
Meatless patties, frozen, Morningstar	38.8	549
Hot dog, turkey links	39.0	495
Sweetbreads, beef, braised	40.0	613
Cheese, Ched-R-Low, Alpine Lace	40.0	640
Combos, cheddar	40.0	1066
Herring, pickled	40.8	595
Bacon, cooked, crumbled	42.0	408
Danish pastry, apple, Sara Lee	42.0	800
Corned beef brisket, cooked	42.6	568
Tongue, pork	42.7	613
Chili, plain, Gebhardt	43.0	530
Sour cream non-dairy substitute	45.0	479
Doughnuts, Hostess Old Fashioned (5)	45.0	850
Tongue, lamb	45.3	624
Frogs' legs, floured, fried	45.3	667
Cheese Whiz	45.6	640
Akee, fresh	46.0	510

Food	Per 8 ozs.	
	Fat grams	Calories
Ham salad, homemade	46.0	574
Lamb loin, lean, broiled	46.0	672
Carnation Chocolate Crunch breakfast bar	46.0	869
Mustard, French's prepared	48.0	288
Sour cream	48.0	496
Cremora, original	48.0	576
Feta cheese, Sargento	48.0	600
Tongue, beef	48.0	642
Beef, T-bone, lean 1/4" charbroiled	48.0	675
Quiche, mushroom, take-out	48.0	683
Cheese Twin, Delicia	48.0	720
Chocolate, Baker's semi-sweet chips	48.0	824
Mustard, Gray Poupon	48.0	864
Falafel	48.0	920
Doughnuts, powdered sugar, Drake's	48.0	960
Shake & Bake, country mild recipe	48.0	1040
Doo Dads	48.0	1120
Tortilla chips, Doritos	48.0	1120
M & Ms	48.0	1144
Pork chop, center loin, broiled	49.0	709
Goose, with skin, roasted	49.6	696
Sweet and sour pork	50.0	940
Mousse, Sara Lee	50.3	770
Beef porterhouse, fat trimmed, broiled	50.6	693
Biscuits, homemade	51.2	1016
Tuna, packed in oil, Starkist	52.0	600
Doughnuts, glazed	52.0	940
Chicken and noodle dinner, Armour	53.0	167
Quiche, cheese, take-out	53.0	755
Doughnuts, cake type	53.0	933
Caramel bar, Little Debbie	55.0	1162
Egg salad, take-out	56.0	614
Egg salad, homemade	57.0	615
Chef's salad, with ham and turkey	58.4	1040
Andes creme de menthe thins	58.5	945
Bratwurst, pork, cooked	59.0	683
Chocolate chip cookies	59.0	987
Beef, ground, regular	60.0	702
Carnation peanut butter/chocolate chip breakfast bar	63.3	1151
Pork sausage, country style, cooked	64.0	384
Sausage, Oscar Mayer	64.0	664
Bologna, beef, Oscar Mayer	64.0	720
Miracle Whip, lite	64.0	720

WATCH OUT — EAT VERY RARELY

Food	Per 8 ozs.	
	Fat grams	Calories
Paté, liver	64.0	720
Cheese, Romano	64.0	880
Tostada, Lance	64.0	1200
Chitterlings pork skins, simmered	65.0	688
Pastrami, beef, thin sliced	66.0	792
Peanut butter cookies	66.0	1153
Quiche Lorraine, take-out	67.0	939
Franks, jumbo cheese, Eckrich	68.0	720
Pie crust, Pillsbury (2 cups)	68.8	1082
Pork spareribs, braised	69.3	901
Hershey's Kisses (48 pieces)	69.6	1224
Peanuts, in oil, Planters	70.0	900
Walnuts, black, chopped, Planters	71.0	759
Nestle's semi-sweet chocolate candy	71.2	1192
Cheese, baby Swiss, Cracker Barrel	72.0	880
Colby cheese, Golden Image cheese substitute	72.0	880
Cheese, blue, Kraft	72.0	880
Cheese, mild cheddar	72.0	912
Chocolate, semi-sweet, baking	72.0	1088
Hershey's chocolate bar	72.3	1239
Walnuts, English halves, Planters	74.0	770
Sesame seeds, dried	75.0	825
Whipped cream	80.0	720
Whipping cream, Land o' Lakes	80.0	720
Cream cheese, Philadelphia	80.0	800
Hot dog, beef links	80.0	880
Mayonnaise type salad dressing	80.0	912
Pork skins, Lance	80.0	1120
Potato chips, Lay's	80.0	1200
Frito's	80.0	1280
Chito's puff balls	80.0	1280
Sausage roll, take-out	82.4	1082
Sausage, pork, Armour	88.0	880
Dressing, Kraft French regular	91.2	944
Touch of Butter, tub	96.0	800
Paté, goose liver, canned	96.0	1048
Cashew nuts, dry-roasted	104.0	1304
Miracle Whip, regular	112.0	1120
Peanuts, dry roasted in the shell	112.0	1280
Spanish peanuts, dry roasted	112.0	1280
Cashew nuts, oil-roasted	112.0	1360
Peanut butter, Skippy super chunky	119.0	1330
Almonds	119.2	1326

WATCH OUT — EAT VERY RARELY

Food	Per 8 ozs.	
	Fat grams	Calories
Chocolate, Baker's unsweetened	120.0	1136
Blue cheese dressing, Kraft	121.6	1216
Nuts, mixed, Eagle	128.0	1440
Pinyon nuts, dried	136.0	1288
Filbert nuts, dried	142.4	1432
Filbert nuts, dry-roasted	150.4	1504
Margarine spread, Parkay (16 Tbls.)	155.2	1408
Pecans, Planter's	160.0	1520
Macadamia nuts	168.0	1680
Blue Bonnet better butter blend, regular	176.0	1440
Butter, stick	184.0	1632
Chicken fat	205.0	1846
Lard (16 Tbls.)	205.0	1849
Olive oil (16 Tbls.)	216.0	1909
Peanut oil (16 Tbls.)	216.0	1909
Canola oil	218.0	1927
Crisco (16 Tbls.)	224.0	1920
Corn oil (16 Tbls.)	224.0	1920
Crisco oil (16 Tbls.)	224.0	1920

EAT VERY RARELY

BIOTECH ALPHABETICAL LISTING OF FOODS

Food	Per 8 ozs.		
	Fat grams	Calories	Color Zone
Acerola juice	7.0	51	YELLOW
Adzuki beans, boiled	2.0	149	GREEN
Akee, fresh	46.0	510	RED
Alaskan crab, canned	2.6	219	YELLOW
Ale, brown, bottled	0.0	66	GREEN
Alfalfa sprouts	0.0	5	GREEN
Allspice	0.0	288	GREEN
Almonds	119.2	1326	RED
Ameranth, box mix	2.8	149	YELLOW
Andes creme de menthe thins	58.5	945	RED
Angelfood cake	0.4	166	GREEN
Anisette, liqueur	0.0	789	GREEN
Apple fruit snack, Weight Watcher's	0.6	800	GREEN
Apple juice, Mott's	0.2	117	GREEN
Apple pie, Banquet	26.6	606	RED
Apple pie, Sara Lee homestyle	38.0	653	RED
Apple, fresh	0.0	81	GREEN
Applebutter, Smucker's	0.0	560	GREEN
Applesauce, sweetened	0.0	194	GREEN
Applesauce, unsweetened	0.0	104	GREEN
Artichoke, plain	0.2	53	GREEN
Asparagus soup with milk	7.9	161	YELLOW
Asparagus, cooked	0.0	60	GREEN
Asparagus, fresh	0.0	60	GREEN
Avocado guacomole dip, Kraft	32.0	400	RED
Avocado, California, fresh	29.8	306	RED
Baby lima beans	0.0	186	GREEN
Bacon bits, Betty Crocker	24.0	600	RED
Bacon bits, Hormel	32.0	480	RED
Bacon bits, Oscar Mayer	32.0	672	RED
Bacon, cooked, crumbled	42.0	408	RED
Baked beans	3.0	120	YELLOW
Baked beans, Campbell's	3.0	240	YELLOW
Baked custard, homemade	14.6	305	YELLOW
Baking powder	0.0	96	GREEN
Baking soda	0.0	240	GREEN
Bamboo shoots, LaChoy	0.0	6	GREEN
Bananas, fresh, whole	0.0	190	GREEN
Barley, cooked	0.6	193	GREEN
Basil seasoning	0.0	144	GREEN
Basil, French's	0.0	144	GREEN
Bay leaf seasoning	0.0	240	GREEN
Bay leaf	0.0	240	GREEN

Food	Per 8 ozs.		
	Fat grams	Calories	Color Zone
Beans and Franks dinner, Banquet	11.2	280	YELLOW
Beans, French, raw	4.0	52	YELLOW
Beans, Great Northern, canned	2.0	180	GREEN
Beans, pink, boiled	0.0	248	GREEN
Beef brains, simmered	28.2	363	RED
Beef chili beans, Chef Boyardee	18.1	352	YELLOW
Beef chuck arm roast, braised	37.8	635	RED
Beef flank steak, lean, raw	2.6	213	YELLOW
Beef heart, simmered	12.8	397	YELLOW
Beef liver	10.6	365	YELLOW
Beef noodles and gravy, Banquet	6.9	206	YELLOW
Beef pepper steak, Healthy Choice	3.4	211	YELLOW
Beef porterhouse, fat trimmed, broiled	50.6	693	RED
Beef pot pie, Morton's	35.4	494	RED
Beef sirloin tip, raw	8.0	240	YELLOW
Beef stew, Chef Boyardee	14.9	251	YELLOW
Beef stroganoff lite dinner, Armour	4.2	178	YELLOW
Beef tenderloin, raw	2.6	187	YELLOW
Beef top round, raw	2.6	213	YELLOW
Beef, chuck roast, lean, raw	5.3	213	YELLOW
Beef, extra lean ground	22.0	404	RED
Beef, eye of the round, raw	5.3	213	YELLOW
Beef, ground, regular	60.0	702	RED
Beef, New York strip	9.1	304	YELLOW
Beef, rib eye, raw	5.3	240	YELLOW
Beef, T-bone, lean 1/4" charbroiled	48.0	675	RED
Beer, Budweiser lite	0.0	73	GREEN
Beer, regular	0.0	96	GREEN
Biscuits, homemade	51.2	1016	RED
Biscuits, mixed with milk	20.8	728	RED
Black beans	0.0	228	GREEN
Blackberries, fresh	0.0	74	GREEN
Blackeyed peas, cooked	0.0	180	GREEN
Bloody Mary mix, with Tabasco	0.9	75	GREEN
Blue Bonnet better butter blend, regular	176.0	1440	RED
Blue cheese dressing, Kraft	121.6	1216	RED
Blueberries, fresh	0.0	82	GREEN
Blueberry pie, Banquet	27.0	655	RED
Bluefin fish, fresh	11.2	325	YELLOW
Bluefish, raw	3.0	240	YELLOW
Bok Choy	0.0	68	GREEN
Bologna, beef, Oscar Mayer	64.0	720	RED
Borage, cooked	2.0	50	GREEN

Food	Per 8 ozs.		
	Fat grams	Calories	Color Zone
Borage, raw	2.0	18	GREEN
Boysenberries, fresh	0.0	62	GREEN
Bran muffins, homemade	32.0	667	RED
Bran, Miller's processed	1.0	186	GREEN
Bran, Quaker Oat	7.6	330	YELLOW
Brandy, fruit flavor	0.0	688	GREEN
Bratwurst, pork, cooked	59.0	683	RED
Brazil nuts	23.2	230	RED
Bread & butter pickles, Vlasic	0.0	240	GREEN
Bread crumbs, soft	1.3	122	GREEN
Bread, white, regular (8 slices)	4.0	480	YELLOW
Breading frying mix	0.0	720	GREEN
Breadsticks, Italian soft	8.0	640	YELLOW
Breadsticks, Oro Wheat cheese	16.0	880	YELLOW
Breadsticks, Stella Dora	8.0	320	YELLOW
Breadsticks, traditional, whole wheat	2.6	160	YELLOW
Broad beans	0.0	186	GREEN
Broccoli, cooked	0.0	44	GREEN
Broccoli, fresh	0.0	24	GREEN
Brussells sprouts, cooked	0.0	40	GREEN
Brussells sprouts, fresh	0.0	40	GREEN
Burdock root, cooked	0.9	110	GREEN
Burdock root, raw	0.9	85	GREEN
Burrito, crisp fried, Van de Camp	20.0	487	YELLOW
Butter beans	0.0	160	GREEN
Butter, stick	184.0	1632	RED
Buttermilk biscuits	12.0	240	YELLOW
Buttermilk	3.5	125	YELLOW
Cabbage, cooked	0.0	4	GREEN
Cabbage, fresh, grated	0.0	5	GREEN
Cabbage, swamp, cooked	0.9	16	GREEN
Cabbage, swamp, raw, chopped	Tr	11	GREEN
Canadian bacon	15.8	356	YELLOW
Candy corn	0.0	824	GREEN
Cannellini beans	0.0	192	GREEN
Canola oil	218.0	1927	RED
Cantaloupe, fresh	0.0	180	GREEN
Caramel bar, Little Debbie	55.0	1162	RED
Caramel corn cakes	0.0	100	GREEN
Cardoon	0.0	51	GREEN
Carnation Chocolate Crunch breakfast bar	46.0	869	RED
Carnation peanut butter/chocolate chip, breakfast	63.3	1151	RED
Carob	7.0	140	YELLOW

Food	Per 8 ozs.		
	Fat grams	Calories	Color Zone
Carp, fresh	12.8	288	YELLOW
Carrots, fresh, shredded	0.0	48	GREEN
Casaba melon	0.0	80	GREEN
Cashew nuts, dry-roasted	104.0	1304	RED
Cashew nuts, oil-roasted	112.0	1360	RED
Cassava root, raw	0.0	274	GREEN
Cauliflower, cooked	0.0	30	GREEN
Cauliflower, fresh	0.0	38	GREEN
Celeriac root (wild celery)	0.0	62	GREEN
Celery, diced, cooked	0.0	20	GREEN
Celery, fresh	0.0	2	GREEN
Champagne	0.0	180	GREEN
Cheese curls, Weight Watcher's	32.0	1120	RED
Cheese Twin, Delicia	48.0	720	RED
Cheese Whiz	45.6	640	RED
Cheese, baby Swiss, Cracker Barrel	72.0	880	RED
Cheese, blue, Kraft	72.0	880	RED
Cheese, Ched-R-Low, Alpine Lace	40.0	640	RED
Cheese, mild cheddar	72.0	912	RED
Cheese, Romano	64.0	880	RED
Cheese, Weight Watcher's sharp cheddar	24.0	560	RED
Chef's salad, with ham and turkey	58.4	1040	RED
Cherries, fresh sweet	0.0	80	GREEN
Cherry pie, Sara Lee homestyle	26.0	540	RED
Chestnuts, roasted	0.4	560	GREEN
Chick peas	4.0	268	YELLOW
Chicken a la King dinner, Armour	4.9	200	YELLOW
Chicken and dumplings, Swanson frozen	11.7	235	YELLOW
Chicken and noodle dinner, Armour	53.0	167	RED
Chicken and noodles, home recipe	18.0	365	YELLOW
Chicken cacciatore, take-out	32.0	525	RED
Chicken dumpling dinner, Banquet	8.0	216	YELLOW
Chicken fat	205.0	1846	RED
Chicken gravy, canned	13.6	192	YELLOW
Chicken noodle soup, Campbell's	2.4	72	YELLOW
Chicken noodles dinner, Banquet	3.2	136	YELLOW
Chicken pot pie, Swanson's	25.1	434	RED
Chicken ravioli, prepared	27.0	693	RED
Chicken, dark meat, no skin, roasted	16.3	424	YELLOW
Chicken, Le Menu, Empress, lite	4.8	203	YELLOW
Chicken, light meat, skinless, roasted	7.2	357	YELLOW
Chicory	0.0	15	GREEN
Chili, plain, Gebhardt	43.0	530	RED

Food	Per 8 ozs.		
	Fat grams	Calories	Color Zone
Chinese cabbage	0.0	10	GREEN
Chinese fried rice, homemade	3.0	206	YELLOW
Chinese noodles, dried	2.0	585	GREEN
Chinese vegetables, LaChoy	0.9	20	GREEN
Chinese water chestnuts	0.9	70	GREEN
Chito's puff balls	80.0	1280	RED
Chitterlings pork skins, simmered	65.0	688	RED
Chives	0.0	16	GREEN
Chocolate chip cookies	59.0	987	RED
Chocolate ice cream	14.4	310	YELLOW
Chocolate ice cream, Baskin Robbins	26.0	528	RED
Chocolate ice cream, Bryers	16.0	320	YELLOW
Chocolate Instant Breakfast with skim milk	0.9	220	GREEN
Chocolate Instant Breakfast with whole milk	8.0	280	YELLOW
Chocolate malted milk	9.0	229	YELLOW
Chocolate milk, 1% fat	2.5	102	YELLOW
Chocolate milk, commercial, 2% fat	5.0	179	YELLOW
Chocolate milk, Hershey's whole milk	9.0	210	YELLOW
Chocolate milk, homemade, 2% milk	5.0	179	YELLOW
Chocolate milk, Land o' Lakes	8.0	210	YELLOW
Chocolate milkshake	6.4	282	YELLOW
Chocolate mocha pie, Weight Watchers	11.6	524	YELLOW
Chocolate mocha, Ultra Slim Fast, skim milk	0.0	200	GREEN
Chocolate pudding, regular	8.0	300	YELLOW
Chocolate, Baker's semi-sweet chips	48.0	824	RED
Chocolate, Baker's unsweetened	120.0	1136	RED
Chocolate, semi-sweet, baking	72.0	1088	RED
Chocolate, Slender	3.2	176	YELLOW
Chow mein, beef, LaChoy	1.3	93	GREEN
Chutney, apple	0.0	656	GREEN
Cider, 6.9% alcohol	0.0	116	GREEN
Cinnamon, ground	0.0	480	GREEN
Clam chowder, New England	2.5	87	YELLOW
Clams, chopped, canned	Tr	110	GREEN
Cloves, seasoning	0.7	110	GREEN
Coca Cola	0.0	93	GREEN
Cocoa, Swiss Miss prepared with milk	1.3	147	GREEN
Coconut, angel flake	2.6	110	YELLOW
Cod, canned	2.0	237	GREEN
Cod, frozen	2.5	293	YELLOW
Coffee, instant	0.0	11	GREEN
Coffee, regular	0.0	4	GREEN
Coffeemate powder	0.9	480	GREEN

| | Per 8 ozs. | | |
Food	Fat grams	Calories	Color Zone
Colby cheese, Golden Image cheese substitute	72.0	880	RED
Cole slaw	3.2	82	YELLOW
Collards	0.0	24	GREEN
Collins mix, Schweppes	0.0	93	GREEN
Combos, cheddar	40.0	1066	RED
Concord grape jellly, S&W	0.0	192	GREEN
Cool Whip cream topping	8.0	224	YELLOW
Corn dogs, Loma Linda	2.0	251	GREEN
Corn muffins	32.0	773	RED
Corn muffins, Dromedary	21.3	640	RED
Corn oil (16 Tbls.)	224.0	1920	RED
Corn pudding, homemade	2.0	194	GREEN
Corn, canned	0.0	206	GREEN
Cornbread, prepared from mix...............................	30.0	987	RED
Corned beef brisket, cooked	42.6	568	RED
Cornmeal, white or yellow	0.0	400	GREEN
Cottage cheese, 1% fat	2.2	162	YELLOW
Cottage cheese, 2% fat	4.4	204	YELLOW
Cow peas, frozen, cooked	0.0	224	GREEN
Crab, Dungeness canned	4.9	199	YELLOW
Crab, raw...	2.6	189	YELLOW
Cracker meal	0.0	400	GREEN
Cranapple juice, Oceanspray	0.0	160	GREEN
Cranberries, fresh...	0.0	54	GREEN
Cranberry beans	0.9	216	GREEN
Cream cheese, Philadelphia	80.0	800	RED
Cream of tartar	0.0	368	GREEN
Cream soda..	0.0	120	GREEN
Creme de menthe liqueur	0.0	992	GREEN
Cremora, original	48.0	576	RED
Crisco (16 Tbls.)..	224.0	1920	RED
Croissant, home recipe	24.0	470	RED
Croissant, Pepperidge Farm	14.0	340	YELLOW
Croutons, Kellogg's	0.0	144	GREEN
Cucumber	0.0	32	GREEN
Cumin seasoning	0.9	384	GREEN
Currants, dried	0.0	408	GREEN
Currants, raw...	0.0	72	GREEN
Curry seasoning	0.9	288	GREEN
Custard, flan, Spanish style with milk	8.0	296	YELLOW
Daiquiri (2)..	0.0	248	GREEN
Dandelion greens, cooked	0.0	34	GREEN
Dandelion greens, raw, chopped	0.0	26	GREEN

Food	Per 8 ozs. Fat grams	Calories	Color Zone
Danish pastry, apple, Sara Lee	42.0	800	RED
Dates, chopped	0.8	489	GREEN
Dates, dried	0.0	912	GREEN
Dock, cooked	0.0	45	GREEN
Doo Dads	48.0	1120	RED
Doughnuts, cake type	53.0	933	RED
Doughnuts, glazed	52.0	940	RED
Doughnuts, Hostess Old Fashioned (5)	45.0	850	RED
Doughnuts, powdered sugar, Drake's	48.0	960	RED
Drambuie liqueur	0.0	880	GREEN
Dressing, fat-free, whipped, Weight Watchers	0.0	258	GREEN
Dressing, Kraft French regular	91.2	944	RED
Dynatrim, chocolate, prepared with 1% milk	4.0	220	YELLOW
Egg noodles	12.0	880	YELLOW
Egg noodles, cooked	2.0	208	GREEN
Egg noodles, Creamette	12.0	884	YELLOW
Egg Pro, regular	8.0	440	YELLOW
Egg salad, homemade	57.0	615	RED
Egg salad, take-out	56.0	614	RED
Eggbeaters egg substitute	0.0	100	GREEN
Eggnog, Carnation lite	8.0	320	YELLOW
Eggplant, fresh, boiled	0.0	26	GREEN
Eggs, raw, medium	24.9	369	RED
Elderberries, raw	0.8	105	GREEN
Enchilada frozen beef dinner, Patio	14.5	314	YELLOW
Enchilada, beef, frozen, Weight Watchers	4.4	167	YELLOW
Enchilada, cheese, frozen, Banquet	6.5	249	YELLOW
Enchilada, chicken, frozen, Banquet	0.4	247	GREEN
Endive	0.0	4	GREEN
English muffins, sourdough	4.0	480	YELLOW
Evaporated milk, Carnation low-fat	4.8	216	YELLOW
Evaporated milk, regular	20.0	338	YELLOW
Evaporated milk, regular	6.0	338	YELLOW
Falafel	48.0	920	RED
Feijoa puree	2.0	119	GREEN
Feijoa, fresh	0.9	114	GREEN
Feta cheese, Sargento	48.0	600	RED
Fettuccine	12.0	880	YELLOW
Fettuccine, prepared	8.0	693	YELLOW
Figs, canned in light syrup	0.0	174	GREEN
Figs, fresh	0.0	74	GREEN
Filbert nuts, dried	142.4	1432	RED
Filbert nuts, dry-roasted	150.4	1504	RED

| | Per 8 ozs. | | |
Food	Fat grams	Calories	Color Zone
Flatfish, cooked	3.5	266	YELLOW
Flavor Tree fruit bears	13.0	891	YELLOW
Flounder, cooked	3.4	266	YELLOW
Flour, arrowroot	0.0	464	GREEN
Flour, bread	0.0	495	GREEN
Flour, cake	0.9	395	GREEN
Fondu, take-out	36.0	606	RED
Franks, big meatless, Loma Linda	22.2	444	RED
Franks, jumbo cheese, Eckrich	68.0	720	RED
Franks, turkey links	24.0	360	RED
French beans, dried	0.9	228	GREEN
French onion dip, Hormel	32.0	440	RED
French toast, Aunt Jemima	10.6	442	YELLOW
French toast, home recipe	14.0	310	YELLOW
French vanilla ice cream, Baskin Robbins	38.0	580	RED
Frito's	80.0	1280	RED
Frogs' legs, floured, fried	45.3	667	RED
Frogs' legs, raw	2.6	168	YELLOW
Fruit cocktail, mixed	0.0	80	GREEN
Fruit salad, water packed	0.0	80	GREEN
Garlic powder seasoning	0.0	192	GREEN
Garlic powder	0.0	288	GREEN
Garlic salt	1.3	144	GREEN
Giblets, capon	12.8	381	YELLOW
Gin, rum, vodka, 100 proof	0.0	698	GREEN
Gin, rum, vodka, 80 proof	0.0	549	GREEN
Gin, rum, vodka, 90 proof	0.0	624	GREEN
Ginger beer	0.0	80	GREEN
Ginger seasoning	0.0	288	GREEN
Ginkgo nuts, canned	0.9	256	GREEN
Ginkgo nuts, raw	0.9	416	GREEN
Gizzards, chicken, simmered	5.0	222	YELLOW
Glazed chicken dinner, Armour	11.9	238	YELLOW
Goose liver	9.6	303	YELLOW
Goose, skinless	28.8	544	RED
Goose, with skin, roasted	49.6	696	RED
Gooseberries, raw	0.8	67	GREEN
Graham crackers (16 crackers)	16.0	960	YELLOW
Grapefruit, fresh	0.0	38	GREEN
Grapes, fresh	0.0	74	GREEN
Gravy, beef, canned	5.6	120	YELLOW
Gravy, brown mix	0.0	8	GREEN
Green beans, snapped, canned	0.0	26	GREEN

Food	Per 8 ozs.		
	Fat grams	Calories	Color Zone
Green peppers, fresh	0.0	38	GREEN
Ground cherries, fresh	0.9	74	GREEN
Ground round	32.0	573	RED
Guava sauce	0.9	86	GREEN
Half and Half, Land o' Lakes	32.0	320	RED
Ham croquettes, home recipe	36.0	560	RED
Ham salad, homemade	46.0	574	RED
Ham steak dinner, Armour	9.5	255	YELLOW
Ham, country cured	29.0	461	RED
Ham, picnic	24.2	312	RED
Handy Pocket cheese sauce/ham, Weight Watchers	12.0	400	YELLOW
Herring, pickled	40.8	595	RED
Herring, raw	20.2	357	RED
Hershey's choc. eclair crunch ice cream bar (2 1/2)	34.6	640	RED
Hershey's chocolate bar	72.3	1239	RED
Hershey's Ice cream sandwich (3)	28.8	672	RED
Hershey's Kisses (48 pieces)	69.6	1224	RED
Hershey's Neo Wave ice cream bar	22.4	512	RED
Hershey's Orange Blossom ice cream bar	16.0	293	YELLOW
Homemade chocolate milk	8.0	208	YELLOW
Homestyle pasta salad with dressing, Kraft	32.0	480	RED
Honey butter, Downey's original	16.0	800	YELLOW
Honey	0.0	773	GREEN
Honeydew, fresh, cubed	0.0	60	GREEN
Hot cocoa mix, Nestle's, 2% milk	6.7	280	YELLOW
Hot dog, beef links	80.0	880	RED
Hot dog, turkey links	39.0	495	RED
Hot fudge topping, Kraft	32.0	1120	RED
Hot roll mix, Pillsbury	16.0	960	YELLOW
Hummus, homemade	21.0	420	RED
Ice pop, lime, Hershey's	0.0	120	GREEN
Iceberg lettuce, shredded	0.0	30	GREEN
Italian pasta salad, take-home	16.0	320	YELLOW
Italian sausage roll, frozen, Ovenstuffs	37.0	857	RED
Jack mackerel, canned, drained	14.4	354	YELLOW
Jackfruit	Tr	160	GREEN
Jam, Smucker's, all flavors	0.0	864	GREEN
Java plum	Tr	82	GREEN
Jello-O, regular	0.0	122	GREEN
Jelly beans	0.6	832	GREEN
Jelly, concord grape, Welch's	0.0	840	GREEN
Juice, body quencher, All Sports	0.0	80	GREEN
Jujube, dried	2.4	640	YELLOW

| | Per 8 ozs. | | |
Food	Fat grams	Calories	Color Zone
Jujube, raw	0.9	184	GREEN
Kale	0.9	40	GREEN
Karo syrup	0.0	960	GREEN
Karo syrup, lite corn	0.0	928	GREEN
Kellogg's Corn Flakes cereal	Tr	88	GREEN
Kellogg's Special K cereal	Tr	83	GREEN
Kelp, raw	1.3	49	GREEN
Ketchup, Heinz	0.0	288	GREEN
Ketchup, low salt, Heinz	0.0	128	GREEN
Kidney beans	0.0	218	GREEN
Kidney beans, canned	0.0	180	GREEN
Kidney, simmered	7.7	325	YELLOW
Kohlrabi, raw	0.0	38	GREEN
Lamb curry, homemade	23.0	460	RED
Lamb loin, lean, broiled	46.0	672	RED
Lamb stew, homemade	7.0	165	YELLOW
Lamb stew, take-out	6.7	165	YELLOW
Lamb sweetbreads, braised	34.6	534	RED
Lard (16 Tbls.)	205.0	1849	RED
Lasagna	4.0	840	YELLOW
Leeks, raw	0.0	64	GREEN
Leg o' lamb, lean, roasted	19.0	432	YELLOW
Lemon curd	0.0	528	GREEN
Lemon Fi-Bar	24.0	720	RED
Lemon ice, Ben & Jerry's	0.0	208	GREEN
Lemon sour mix, Schweppes	0.0	100	GREEN
Lentils	0.0	232	GREEN
Lime juice	0.0	66	GREEN
Lobster Newburg	37.0	464	RED
Lobster, northern, cooked	0.0	220	GREEN
Log Cabin syrup, buttered	0.6	848	GREEN
Log Cabin syrup, lite	0.9	488	GREEN
Loganberries	0.0	90	GREEN
Lotus seed	4.8	752	YELLOW
M & Ms	48.0	1144	RED
Macadamia nuts	168.0	1680	RED
Macaroni and cheese, take out	24.1	406	RED
Macaroni salad, take out	11.4	366	YELLOW
Macaroni	4.0	840	YELLOW
Macaroni, cooked	0.9	197	GREEN
Mandarin orange-flavored drink, Koala	0.0	55	GREEN
Mango, fruit, diced	0.6	109	GREEN
Margarine spread, Parkay (16 Tbls.)	155.2	1408	RED

Food	Per 8 ozs.		
	Fat grams	Calories	Color Zone
Marshmallows, Kraft	0.0	560	GREEN
Mayonnaise type salad dressing	80.0	912	RED
Mayonnaise, home recipe	24.0	100	RED
Meatless patties, frozen, Morningstar	38.8	549	RED
Meatless swiss steak with gravy, Loma Linda	24.6	431	RED
Melon balls, frozen	Tr	55	GREEN
Mexican style dinner, Banquet	12.4	298	YELLOW
Milk, 1%	2.5	158	YELLOW
Milk, 2%	5.0	180	YELLOW
Milk, imitation	8.0	150	YELLOW
Milk, skim	0.4	86	GREEN
Milk, Vitamite, Deihl	5.0	100	YELLOW
Milk, whole, 3.3% fat	8.1	14	YELLOW
Milkshake, vanilla	7.1	265	YELLOW
Miracle Whip, fat-free	0.0	320	GREEN
Miracle Whip, lite	64.0	720	RED
Miracle Whip, regular	112.0	1120	RED
Miso paste	16.0	570	YELLOW
Mixed fruit, water packed	0.0	112	GREEN
Mixed vegetables, canned, Hanover	0.0	220	GREEN
Mixed vegetables, homemade	0.9	78	GREEN
Mixed vegetables, Libby's	0.0	80	GREEN
Molasses, blackstrap	0.0	640	GREEN
Molasses, Brer Rabbit, black and white	0.0	960	GREEN
Molasses, Grandma's Green or Gold label	0.9	1120	GREEN
Moth beans, cooked	3.0	70	YELLOW
Mousse, Sara Lee	50.3	770	RED
Mozzarella cheese substitute	24.0	560	RED
Muffins, blueberry, home recipe	27.0	720	RED
Mulberries	0.9	61	GREEN
Mungo beans, boiled	0.0	190	GREEN
Mungo beans, sprouted seeds, raw	0.0	32	GREEN
Mushrooms, fresh	0.0	29	GREEN
Mushrooms, sauteed with 1 Tbls. margarine	7.0	60	YELLOW
Mustard greens, fresh, boiled	0.0	22	GREEN
Mustard, French's prepared	48.0	288	RED
Mustard, Gray Poupon	48.0	864	RED
Nacho cheese dip, Kraft	32.0	440	RED
Natto	19.4	374	YELLOW
Navy beans, boiled	0.9	258	GREEN
Nestle's Quik chocolate powder	10.6	960	YELLOW
Nestle's Quik chocolate with 2% milk	5.0	210	YELLOW
Nestle's ready-to-drink Quik	9.0	230	YELLOW

Food	Per 8 ozs.		
	Fat grams	Calories	Color Zone
Nestle's semi-sweet chocolate candy	71.2	1192	RED
Nibbles, cherry and chocolate	35.0	1028	RED
Noodles, egg/spinach	8.0	836	YELLOW
Nutra shake, chocolate	12.0	400	YELLOW
Nutri Balance frozen chocolate pudding	16.0	450	YELLOW
Nutri Grain apple breakfast bar	30.8	923	RED
Nuts, mixed, Eagle	128.0	1440	RED
Okra, fresh cooked	0.0	68	GREEN
Olive loaf, Loma Linda	24.0	476	RED
Olive oil (16 Tbls.)	216.0	1909	RED
Olives, ripe	24.0	240	RED
Omelette, Chefwich cheese	27.2	608	RED
Onion ring mix	0.0	800	GREEN
Onions, fresh green	0.0	48	GREEN
Onions, fresh white	0.0	50	GREEN
Orange drink, powder, prepared with water	0.0	115	GREEN
Orange juice, fresh squeezed	0.4	112	GREEN
Orange juice, Minutemaid	0.0	110	GREEN
Orange marmalade, S&W	0.0	192	GREEN
Orange sherbet	4.0	270	YELLOW
Orange, fresh	0.0	96	GREEN
Oyster crackers	8.0	240	YELLOW
Oysters, eastern, canned	16.8	157	YELLOW
Pancake and waffle syrup, Aunt Jemima	0.0	880	GREEN
Pancake and waffle syrup, Golden Griddle	0.0	885	GREEN
Pancake/waffle syrup, lite, Aunt Jemima	0.0	400	GREEN
Papaya, fresh pulp	0.0	80	GREEN
Paprika seasoning	0.0	96	GREEN
Parsnips, raw	0.0	100	GREEN
Passion fruit juice	Tr	126	GREEN
Pasta salad with vegetables	9.1	320	YELLOW
Pasta salad, Lite Italian, with dressing, Kraft	6.0	260	YELLOW
Pasta shell, dried, Mueller's	0.1	840	GREEN
Pastromi, beef, thin sliced	66.0	792	RED
Paté, goose liver, canned	96.0	1048	RED
Paté, liver	64.0	720	RED
Pate, chicken liver, canned	32.0	1904	RED
Peaches, Del Monte, heavy syrup	0.0	180	GREEN
Peanut butter cookies	66.0	1153	RED
Peanut butter, Skippy super chunky	119.0	1330	RED
Peanut oil (16 Tbls.)	216.0	1909	RED
Peanuts, dry roasted in the shell	112.0	1280	RED
Peanuts, in oil, Planters	70.0	900	RED

Food	Per 8 ozs. Fat grams	Calories	Color Zone
Pear, Balsam, raw	0.0	15	GREEN
Pears, fresh	0.0	97	GREEN
Peas and carrots, homemade	0.9	96	GREEN
Peas, pigeon, fresh cooked	3.5	125	YELLOW
Peas, snow	0.0	68	GREEN
Pecans, Planter's	160.0	1520	RED
Pepper	0.9	240	GREEN
Peppermint Schnapps, liqueur	0.0	661	GREEN
Pepperoni pizza, Celeste	34.3	640	RED
Perch, cooked	2.6	264	YELLOW
Pheasant	6.4	235	YELLOW
Phyllo dough	17.0	815	YELLOW
Pickles, sweet gerkin	0.9	320	GREEN
Pickles, zesty dill spears	0.0	32	GREEN
Pie crust, Pillsbury (2 cups)	68.8	1082	RED
Pierogi, cheese	5.3	583	YELLOW
Pierogi, onion	0.6	480	GREEN
Pigs' ears	25.9	396	RED
Pigs' feet	5.0	395	YELLOW
Pike, northern, cooked	5.0	261	YELLOW
Pimientos	0.0	60	GREEN
Pina colada	3.0	349	YELLOW
Pineapple juice, Bluebird, 100% pure juice	0.0	100	GREEN
Pineapple, fresh	0.0	76	GREEN
Pinto beans, frozen, cooked	0.0	405	GREEN
Pinto beans, Green Giant, canned	2.0	180	GREEN
Pinyon nuts, dried	136.0	1288	RED
Pistachio nuts, dry roasted	30.8	368	RED
Pitanga	0.6	57	GREEN
Pizza, Celeste supreme	34.6	613	RED
Pizza, cheese, Kid Cuisine	14.0	444	YELLOW
Pizza, French bread and cheese, Healthy Choice	3.0	408	YELLOW
Plums, fresh sliced	0.9	91	GREEN
Plums, whole, canned	0.0	270	GREEN
Poi	0.0	268	GREEN
Pokeberry shoots, fresh, cooked	0.0	32	GREEN
Polish kielbasa, Mr. Turkey	35.0	472	RED
Pollack, raw	2.0	208	GREEN
Pomelo, raw	0.0	71	GREEN
Popcorn with oil and salt (17 cups)	34.0	697	RED
Popcorn, hot-air popped	3.0	369	YELLOW
Popped corncakes, cheddar	0.0	100	GREEN
Pork chop, center loin, broiled	49.0	709	RED

	Per 8 ozs.		
Food	Fat grams	Calories	Color Zone
Pork chop, lean with fat	34.3	619	RED
Pork liver	10.6	376	YELLOW
Pork sausage, country style, cooked	64.0	384	RED
Pork skins, Lance	80.0	1120	RED
Pork spareribs, braised	69.3	901	RED
Postum, instant, prepared	0.9	14	GREEN
Potato chips, Lay's	80.0	1200	RED
Potato, plain baked	0.0	218	GREEN
Potatoes, peeled, grated	0.0	4	GREEN
Poultry seasoning	0.9	288	GREEN
Pound cake	20.1	351	RED
Pretzels, Shearer's	0.0	320	GREEN
Prunes, canned, heavy syrup	0.0	248	GREEN
Prunes, dried	1.0	380	GREEN
Pudding, Jell-O instant butterscotch	10.0	336	YELLOW
Pudding, Swiss Miss chocolate prepared	12.0	60	YELLOW
Pumpkin pie spice	0.9	288	GREEN
Pumpkin, canned	0.0	70	GREEN
Pumpkin, raw, cubed	0.0	30	GREEN
Purslane, cooked	Tr	21	GREEN
Purslane, raw	Tr	7	GREEN
Quail breast, no skin	8.0	276	YELLOW
Quail breast, with skin	37.1	442	RED
Quaker oatmeal, cooked	2.0	145	GREEN
Quaker puffed wheat (8 cups)	0.0	800	GREEN
Quiche Lorraine, take-out	67.0	939	RED
Quiche, cheese, take-out	53.0	755	RED
Quiche, mushroom, take-out	48.0	683	RED
Radish, fresh	0.0	17	GREEN
Ranch, free salad dressing, Kraft	0.0	260	GREEN
Raspberries, red, fresh	0.0	60	GREEN
Raspberries, red, frozen	0.0	258	GREEN
Raspberry sorbet, Dole	0.0	220	GREEN
Ravioli with beef	8.0	900	YELLOW
Red beans, cooked	0.0	224	GREEN
Refried beans	0.0	260	GREEN
Relish, sweet, Vlasic	0.0	240	GREEN
Rhubarb	1.0	60	GREEN
Rhubarb, frozen	0.9	120	GREEN
Rice Chex cereal, Ralston	0.0	240	GREEN
Rice pudding	8.0	310	YELLOW
Rice, white, cooked	0.6	264	GREEN
Rigatoni, prepared	10.4	533	YELLOW

Food	Per 8 ozs.		
	Fat grams	Calories	Color Zone
Ritz crackers	4.0	476	YELLOW
Roll, submarine	3.4	263	YELLOW
Rose apple, fresh	0.9	73	GREEN
Rosemary, dried	0.9	192	GREEN
Rutabaga, raw	0.0	50	GREEN
Rykrisp	16.0	540	YELLOW
Sage	0.9	96	GREEN
Salisbury steak with gravy, Banquet	21.7	297	RED
Salmon	14.4	833	YELLOW
Salsa, Chi Chi's mild	0.6	72	GREEN
Salsa, chunky mild, Rosarita	1.3	133	GREEN
Salsa, Ortega medium green chili	0.0	96	GREEN
Salt seasoning	1.0	192	GREEN
Saltine crackers (64)	10.6	132	YELLOW
Sardines	26.2	457	RED
Sauerkraut, canned	0.0	56	GREEN
Sausage roll, take-out	82.4	1082	RED
Sausage, Oscar Mayer	64.0	664	RED
Sausage, pork, Armour	88.0	880	RED
Scallops	2.6	185	YELLOW
Scone, plain	32.0	827	RED
Scrambled eggs, Kid Cuisine	33.1	527	RED
Seaweed, dried, Agar	2.6	693	YELLOW
Sesame seeds, dried	75.0	825	RED
Sesbania flowers	Tr	5	GREEN
Sesbania flowers, cooked	Tr	23	GREEN
Shake & Bake, country mild recipe	48.0	1040	RED
Shake and Bake, chicken	32.0	1200	RED
Shake and Bake, fish	16.0	1184	YELLOW
Shake and Bake, pork	16.0	1280	YELLOW
Sharps non-alcoholic beer	0.0	34	GREEN
Shellie beans	0.0	74	GREEN
Sherbet, lime	2.0	260	GREEN
Sherry	0.0	280	GREEN
Shoestring potatoes, Ore Ida	8.0	400	YELLOW
Shrimp creole dinner, Amour	1.0	185	GREEN
Shrimp, steamed	2.4	224	YELLOW
Sirloin strip style dinner, Jaclyn's	4.0	172	YELLOW
Sloe gin	0.0	661	GREEN
Soft drink, 7-Up, diet	0.0	0	GREEN
Soft drink, club soda	0.0	0	GREEN
Soft drink, Fresca	0.0	4	GREEN
Sole, cooked	3.4	264	YELLOW

Food	Per 8 ozs. Fat grams	Calories	Color Zone
Sole, raw	2.6	205	YELLOW
Soup, clam chowder, Manhattan	0.6	66	GREEN
Sour cream non-dairy substitute	45.0	479	RED
Sour cream	48.0	496	RED
Soy sauce	0.0	120	GREEN
Spaghetti sauce, Prego	10.0	260	YELLOW
Spaghetti sauce, Ragu thick and zesty	23.8	222	RED
Spaghetti sauce, Ragu, meatless	10.0	180	YELLOW
Spaghetti	4.0	840	YELLOW
Spanish peanuts, dry roasted	112.0	1280	RED
Spinach, cooked	0.0	0	GREEN
Spinach, fresh	0.0	1	GREEN
Strawberries, fresh	0.0	45	GREEN
Strawberry ice cream	10.0	232	YELLOW
Strawberry ice cream, Bryers	6.0	220	YELLOW
Strawberry jam, S&W	0.0	192	GREEN
Strawberry sorbet	0.6	142	GREEN
Stuffing, Brownberry	2.5	200	YELLOW
Succotash, homemade	2.0	204	GREEN
Succotash, S&W country style	2.0	204	GREEN
Sugar apple, fresh, cut up	3.0	236	YELLOW
Sugar Twin, white and brown	0.0	96	GREEN
Sugar, brown, packed	0.0	821	GREEN
Sugar, white, granulated	0.0	770	GREEN
Sunkist funfruit	0.9	89	GREEN
Swedish meatballs with sauce, Dining Delight	8.8	249	YELLOW
Sweet and sour pork	50.0	940	RED
Sweet potato, canned in syrup	Tr	183	GREEN
Sweet potato, fresh, mashed	0.9	344	GREEN
Sweetbreads, beef, braised	40.0	613	RED
Sweetbreads, veal, braised	32.0	581	RED
Swiss chard, cooked	0.9	36	GREEN
Swiss chard, fresh	0.9	6	GREEN
Swordfish, raw	9.0	275	YELLOW
Syrup, Weight Watchers	0.0	400	GREEN
Tamales with sauce, Van Camps	16.0	293	YELLOW
Tamales, beef, frozen, Banquet	13.0	305	YELLOW
Tamales, Wolf brand	27.0	350	RED
Tamarind, fresh, cut up	0.9	287	GREEN
Tangerine, fresh	Tr	86	GREEN
Tapioca	8.0	290	YELLOW
Taro, cooked	0.9	188	GREEN
Taro, raw sliced	0.9	112	GREEN

Food	Per 8 ozs.		
	Fat grams	Calories	Color Zone
Tea, amaretto, Celestial regular tea	Tr	3	GREEN
Tea, cinnamon stick, regular, Bigelow	Tr	1	GREEN
Tea, cinnamon, apple spice, Celestial	Tr	3	GREEN
Tea, orange, spice, herbal, Bigelow	Tr	1	GREEN
Tempeh	12.0	320	YELLOW
Tequilla Sunrise	0.1	252	GREEN
Three Musketeers, chocolate bar	30.5	990	RED
Tofu, Mori-Nu extra firm	4.6	137	YELLOW
Tofu, Mori-Nu firm	6.0	137	YELLOW
Tofu, Mori-Nu soft	6.0	122	YELLOW
Tofu, regular	12.0	176	YELLOW
Tofu, Spring Creek barbecue baked	16.0	352	YELLOW
Tomatillo, fresh	0.9	42	GREEN
Tomato juice	0.2	41	GREEN
Tomato soup, Campbell's condensed	4.0	140	YELLOW
Tomato, fresh	0.0	26	GREEN
Tongue, beef	48.0	642	RED
Tongue, lamb	45.3	624	RED
Tongue, pork	42.7	613	RED
Tonic water	0.0	85	GREEN
Tortilla chips, Doritos	48.0	1120	RED
Tostada, Lance	64.0	1200	RED
Touch of Butter, tub	96.0	800	RED
Tree fern, chopped, cooked	0.9	56	GREEN
Triple Sec	0.0	632	GREEN
Trout	12.5	312	YELLOW
Tuna melt, Chefwich	22.4	576	RED
Tuna salad, take-out	19.0	383	YELLOW
Tuna, packed in oil, Starkist	52.0	600	RED
Tuna, packed in water	8.0	360	YELLOW
Turkey giblets	11.2	389	YELLOW
Turkey gizzards, simmered	6.0	236	YELLOW
Turkey pastrami, thin sliced	11.6	276	YELLOW
Turkey pot pie, Swanson's	24.0	434	RED
Turkey, ground, fresh	16.0	320	YELLOW
Turkey, ground, fried	16.0	320	YELLOW
Turnip greens, cooked	0.0	48	GREEN
Turnip greens, raw	Tr	36	GREEN
Turnip greens, raw, frozen	Tr	34	GREEN
Ultra Slim chocolate pudding, prepared	0.9	200	GREEN
Ultra Slim Fast, French vanilla, prepared	Tr	220	GREEN
Ultra Slim Fast, French vanilla, skim milk	Tr	190	GREEN
V-8 Juice	0.2	53	GREEN

Food	Per 8 ozs.		
	Fat grams	Calories	Color Zone
Vanilla ice cream, Baskin Robbins	28.0	480	RED
Vanilla ice cream, Bryers	16.0	300	YELLOW
Vanilla ice cream, regular	14.4	268	YELLOW
Vanilla ice cream, rich	23.6	350	RED
Vanilla wafers, Murray	24.0	64	RED
Veal parmigiana	34.2	531	RED
Vega burger, Loma Linda	2.0	220	GREEN
Vegetable soup, Campbell's condensed	2.0	90	GREEN
Vegetable with chicken pot pie, Morton's	32.0	480	RED
Vermicelli	4.0	840	YELLOW
Vinegar, Regina, red wine	0.0	32	GREEN
Vinegar, Whitehouse apple cider	0.0	16	GREEN
Waffles, buttermilk, frozen, Aunt Jemima	19.2	573	YELLOW
Waffles, Eggo frozen buttermilk	29.0	756	RED
Waffles, Eggo frozen homestyle	29.0	756	RED
Waffles, frozen, Multi-Grain, Weight Watchers	21.3	640	RED
Waffles, mix prepared with egg and milk	24.6	631	RED
Waffles, Special K	0.0	320	GREEN
Walnuts, black, chopped, Planters	71.0	759	RED
Walnuts, English halves, Planters	74.0	770	RED
Watercress, chopped	Tr	2	GREEN
Watercress, chopped	0.9	4	GREEN
Watermelon	0.0	52	GREEN
Wheat germ, plain, toasted	12.0	431	YELLOW
Whipped cream	80.0	720	RED
Whipping cream, Land o' Lakes	80.0	720	RED
White beans	1.0	254	GREEN
White bread, Schwebel's (6 slices)	8.0	560	YELLOW
Wine, dessert sweet, 18.8% alcohol	0.0	363	GREEN
Wine, dessert, dry 18.8% alcohol	0.0	299	GREEN
Wine, sweet	0.0	356	GREEN
Winged beans, cooked	10.0	252	YELLOW
Yam, cubed, cooked	0.9	158	GREEN
Yambean, boiled	0.0	110	GREEN
Yams, candied, canned	0.9	360	GREEN
Yardlong beans	0.0	204	GREEN
Yeast, brewer's dried	0.9	400	GREEN
Yellow beans	0.0	44	GREEN
Yellowtail	12.0	330	YELLOW
Yogurt, all flavors, Cabot	3.0	110	YELLOW
Yogurt, apple, Yoplait original	4.0	480	YELLOW
Yogurt, Ben & Jerry's frozen cherry	9.6	320	YELLOW
Yogurt, blueberry, non-fat lite, Dannon	0.0	109	GREEN

Food	Per 8 ozs.		
	Fat grams	Calories	Color Zone
Yogurt, blueberry, Yoplait original	8.0	240	YELLOW
Yogurt, frozen, all flavors, Bressler's gourmet	3.2	232	YELLOW
Yogurt, frozen, all flavors, Bressler's	3.2	216	YELLOW
Yogurt, frozen, TCBY	2.0	220	GREEN
Yogurt, low-fat, fruit	2.6	225	YELLOW
Yogurt, non-fat	0.4	127	GREEN
Yogurt, plain, regular	7.4	138	YELLOW
Yogurt, Weight Watchers, all flavors	0.0	90	GREEN
Zucchini squash, breaded, Ore Ida	21.0	400	RED
Zucchini squash, cooked	1.3	20	GREEN
Zucchini squash, cooked	0.0	28	GREEN
Zucchini squash, fresh	0.0	28	GREEN
Zucchini squash, Italian style	0.9	28	GREEN
Zucchini squash, raw sliced	0.9	28	GREEN

LOW-FAT FOODS TO SUBSTITUTE FOR HIGH-FAT FOODS

The following chart will help you make good low-fat food choices. Be sure to follow these guidelines when dining out or preparing meals at home. Just following these suggestions will likely give you a good start on a weight management program.

Instead of this:	Fat grams	Try this:	Fat grams	
Dark meat chicken	16	White meat chicken	5	
Dark meat turkey	12	White meat turkey	3	
Lamb chop	14	Veal cutlet (3 oz.)	4	
Tuna, oil packed	7	Tuna, water packed	1/2	
Salmon	9	Halibut	3	or
		Crab	1	or
		Lobster	1/2	or
		Clams	2	or
		Scallops	1	or
		Shrimp, boiled	1	

Instead of this:	Fat grams	Try this:	Fat grams	
Ground beef	20	Vegetarian burger	2	or
		Chef Edward's Special Recipe	4	
Chuck roast	19	Braised brisket	10	or
		Bottom round roast	6	
Sirloin	17	T-bone	10	or
		Top Round	4	
Eggs with yolks	5	Eggs, whites only	0	
		(or Egg Beater-type product)		
Beef or chicken liver	8	Simmered kidney	3	
Pork chops	14	Pork tenderloin	5	
Pork roast	28			
Pork shoulder	26			
Pork spareribs	30			
Whole milk	9	Skim milk	1/2	
Whole milk yogurt	4	Skim milk yogurt	0	
Pork sausage	8	Beef or vegetarian bacon	2	or
		ground turkey	2	
Hot dogs	16	Turkey dogs	8	or
		Vegetarian dogs	3	
Luncheon meats	8	95% fat-free luncheon meats	1	
Butter	12	Sunflower or low-fat margarine	4	
Sauces	27	Vegetable or fruit juices	0	
Oils	13	Stock pot flavorings, vegetable oil sprays	0	
Chocolate	13	Carob flavor mix powder	0	
Cream soups	12	Chicken noodle soup	3	
Sour cream	3	Light sour cream	1	or
		lowfat yogurt	0	
Chocolate chips	14	Raisins	1/2	
Cheddar cheese	12	Part-skim mozzarella	5	
Ice cream	15	Sherbet, ice milk, frozen lowfat yogurt	2	
Baked potato with butter & sour cream	15	Baked potato with stone ground mustard &/or salsa	0	
Cream	4	Skim milk	0	or
		Low-fat, non-dairy substitute	1	

Instead of this:	Fat grams	Try this:	Fat grams	
Bacon bits	10	Fresh chives	0	
Cottage cheese	5	Low-fat cottage cheese	2	
Potato chips	10	Air popped popcorn	0	
Cream cheese	10	Fat-free ricotta cheese	1	
Nuts	15	Water chestnuts	0	
		Roasted chestnuts	0	
Mayonnaise	11	Non-fat mayonnaise	3	or
		non-fat yogurt with mustard		
		or vinegar	0	
Oil-type salad dressing	9	Fat-free dressing	1	
Sauces or gravies	15	Chef Edward's Gourmet Sauces	0	

FOODS YOU CAN EAT AS MUCH AS YOU WANT

Yes, it's true. There are many foods that you can eat whenever you like, and as much as you want. (Within reason, please. Nobody really needs to eat 20 baked potatoes.)

While it sounds illogical, the best way to lose weight is to eat whenever you are genuinely hungry, as long as you eat the right foods.

Let's face it - severe hunger, such as when counting calories or otherwise reducing food intake, leads one to binge eating. After a while, hunger becomes so strong that a person eats larger amounts of food. And usually, the food is the wrong kind, such as fat-laden snack foods, pizza or some other high-fat food.

The way to lose weight is this - eat food when you get hungry, but eat the right foods. Eat small snacks throughout the day. A constant supply of food keeps the metabolism high and actually accelerates a weight management program.

When you get hungry, reach for those carrots, celery, apples, oranges or complex carbohydrates. You'll feel satisfied, you'll look great and you'll feel supercharged with energy.

To help you pick the right foods, here's a list of what you should eat between meals throughout the day if you get hungry. If you center your main meals around these foods, you'll absolutely power-charge your weight program and feel great at the same time!

FOODS TO EAT WHEN YOU GET HUNGRY

VEGETABLES

Artichoke
Asparagus *
Bamboo shoots *
Beets *
Broccoli *
Cabbage *
Carrots *
Cauliflower *
Celery *
Chives *
Cucumber *
Eggplant *
Endive *
Fennel *
Green Beans *
Horseradish *
Kale *
Leeks *
Lettuce *
Mung beans *
Mushrooms *
Okra *
Onion *
Parsley *
Parsnips *
Peas
Peppers, green, sweet or hot *
Pickles, dill or sour *
Pumpkin *
Red Radish *
Rhubarb *
Sauerkraut *
Shallots *
Snap Beans *
Spinach *
Squash *
Swiss Chard *

VEGETABLES (continued)

Watercress *
Wax beans *
Zucchini *
Tomatoes or tomato juice *
Turnip *
Water chestnuts *

CARBOHYDRATES

Corn
Black beans
Kidney beans
Grains
Potatoes
Rice

FRUITS

Apples
Bananas
Grapefruit
Lemon
Mandarin
Mango
Oranges
Papaya
Pineapple
Raspberries
Strawberries

MISCELLANEOUS

Coffee *
Tea *
Noodle soup *

NEGATIVE CALORIE FOODS

The foods listed with an asterisk after them are very low-calorie foods. They contain less than 30 calories per serving. As you can see, almost all the low-calorie foods are vegetables, and almost all vegetables are low-calorie foods.

These low-calorie foods have sometimes been called "negative calorie" foods. The reasoning behind calling them this is rather simple. The physical act of eating burns up 1.5 calories per minute. Since a serving of one of the above foods contains less than 30 calories, all of the calories in the food will be burned up by the body within 20 minutes. Assuming that the time spent eating a meal averages 30 minutes or so, it is actually possible to eat a serving of any of the low-calorie foods and burn up more calories than the food contains before the meal is over!

A person could eat several servings of these low-calorie foods at every meal and not gain weight. The calories would be completely used up long before the next meal. They would likely lose weight rather quickly since all of the low-calorie foods are also very low in fat content.

An additional benefit of the low-calorie foods is that they are nutritionally dense. These foods are low in calories, yet high in nutrition. They are loaded with vitamins, minerals and antioxidants, such as beta carotene. High-fat foods, on the other hand, are not nutritionally dense. They are high in calories but low in nutrition. Eating the low-calorie nutritionally dense foods not only superpowers your weight management program, it can also boost your imune system and help you feel healthier.

Important – normal daily activity burns up 2.6 calories per minute, while any active sport or exercise burns up 5–15 calories per minute. So if a large portion of your daily food intake is composed of the nutrient-dense 1.5-calorie-per-minute foods, your weight management plan will be greatly improved. This is because your body will need to rely on stored fat for fuel since you are eating low–calorie, low–fat foods. The end result – you will lose weight more easily, more quickly and more permanently than with most other "diet" plans.

HOW TO CALCULATE YOUR OWN METABOLISM

It is possible to calculate your own individual metabolic rate. This daily metabolic rate, called the basal metabolism, is the number of calories burned up by your body for normal body functions. These are the calories required every day to keep your heart, lungs, muscles, organs and autonomic system functioning. It is also quite easy to factor in the additional calories that you burn based on your physical activity.

Knowing your own basal metabolism will enable you to custom-design a weight management program specifically for you. Your weight loss will then likely be greatly accelerated without the drastic lifestyle changes required by most diets.

The formula, called the Harris–Benedict formula, has been used by professional nutritionists for years as the most authoritative way to calculate basal metabolism.

THE HARRIS–BENEDICT FORMULA FOR MEN

1. Multiply height in inches by 2.54 to determine height in centimeters.

2. Multiply height in centimeters by 5.0 to determine the calories needed for body height.

3. Divide weight in pounds by 2.2 to determine weight in kilograms.

4. Multiply weight in kilograms by 13.7 to determine the calories needed for body weight.

5. Multiply age by 6.8 to determine the age factor number.

6. Determine physical activity level number:
   Low activity level   – 1.3
   Normal activity level   – 1.4
   High activity level   – 1.5

7. Total Basal Metabolism = 66 + calories needed for height + calories needed for weight - age factor number x activity level number.

Let's work through a real–life example to see how it works. Let's calculate the basal metabolism for a 35 year old man, 6'0" tall, weighing 200 pounds.

1. 72 inches x 2.54 = 182.88 centimeters

2. 182.88 x 5.0 = 914 calories needed for height

3. 200 pounds divided by 2.2 = 90.9 kilograms

4. 90.9 kilograms x 13.7 = 1245 calories needed for weight

5. 35 years x 6.8 = 238 age factor

6. Normal physical activity number of 1.4

7. 66 + 914 + 1245 - 238 x 1.4 = 2781 calories needed per day

This is a good number of calories for a man. If he centers his meals around low-fat foods, his weight management program will be successful, and he will be able to eat large quantities of satisfying, good-tasting food.

THE HARRIS–BENEDICT FORMULA FOR WOMEN

1. Multiply height in inches by 2.54 to determine height in centimeters.

2. Multiply height in centimeters by 1.7 to determine the calories needed for body height.

3. Divide weight in pounds by 2.2 to determine weight in kilograms.

4. Multiply weight in kilograms by 9.6 to determine the calories needed for body weight.

5. Multiply age by 4.7 to determine the age factor number.

6. Determine the physical activity level number:
   Low activity level   1.3
   Normal activity level 1.4
   High activity level   1.5

7. Total Basal Metabolism = 665 + calories needed for height + calories needed for weight - age factor number x activity level number.

Now let's calculate the basal metabolism for a 35 year-old woman, 5'2" tall, weighing 125 pounds.

1. 62 inches x 2.54 = 157.48 centimeters

2. 157.48 x 1.7 = 267 calories needed for height

3. 125 pounds divided by 2.2 = 56.81 kilograms

4. 56.81 x 9.6 = 545 calories needed for weight

5. 35 years x 4.7 = 164.5 age factor

6. Normal physical activity number of 1.4

7. 665 + 267 + 545 -164.5 x 1.4 = 1837 calories needed per day

The woman in our example needs to eat 1837 calories per day just to maintain her present weight. This is actually a fairly high level of calories per day for a woman. She will have no trouble eating large portions of good food without gaining weight.

Take the time right now to calculate your own basal metabolism using the Harris-Benedict Formula. Knowing your personal basal metabolism may give you an indication why previous "diets" have not worked for you. As we've already discussed, fat calories are not the same as protein or carbohydrate calories. Fat calories are not nutritionally dense, and contain about twice the calories per gram of protein or carbohydrates. This is why many diets fail for many people time and time again – the diets do not take into account the difference between fat and other calories.

An especially appealing aspect of the Biotech Plan is that you do not need to count calories to achieve maximum weight loss. The entire program has been designed around the proven low-fat method. Rather than counting calories, learn to concentrate instead on eating low-fat foods. Most low-fat foods will also be nutritionally dense, thus giving you good nutrition. They will also contain more fiber than fatty foods. The combination of high fiber and needed nutrients will fill you up and help you stay healthier.

The effort that you spend learning to eat the Biotech low-fat way will be far surpassed by its many benefits. And your body will love you for it. Happy eating!

NUTRITIONAL VALUES FOR BIOTECH RECIPES

L isted below are all the recipes included in this book. The corresponding figures in the columns indicate the calories, fat grams and percent of fat per serving.

Some items look like they contain a high percentage of fat, such as some of the marinades, stocks and sauces. Be sure to look at the entire recipe when making your choices. For instance, the champagne balsamic vinaigrette gets 46% of its calories from fat, but it only contains .6 grams of fat. It's so low in calories that it makes it look like it's higher in fat when that really isn't the case.

Remember too that marinades and sauces are added to other entrees. Increasing the volume of food eaten with a sauce decreases the fat percentage tremendously.

Use this chart if you need to find a meal to fit into a calorie or fat-gram requirement that you may have. It will help you make the proper choices.

RECIPE	CAL	FAT GM	FAT %
ANGEL FOOD ALMOND CAKE	78	0	0
CHEF EDWARD'S SALTLESS TABLE SEASONING	1	0	5
YOGURT CREAM SAUCE	31	.1	3
ROASTED RED PEPPER SAUCE	13	.1	6

RECIPE	CAL	FAT GM	FAT %
CRANBERRY APPLE RELISH	43	.1	1
PINEAPPLE CHUTNEY	23	.1	3
SHALLOT RASPBERRY CHUTNEY	29	.1	3
STRAWBERRY CHEESE	72	.1	1
QUICK AND EASY MARINADE	30	.1	2
SEAFOOD MARINADE	35	.2	3
BASIC BEEF STOCK	12	.2	12
CAJUN REMOULADE SAUCE	28	.2	5
BAKED ACORN SQUASH	144	.2	1
RASPBERRY CINNAMON COULIS	30	.2	7
SMOKED TOMATO SALSA	23	.3	9
OVEN JERKED FRENCH FRIES	99	.4	3
PARMESAN AND DILL DIP	24	.4	15
PIZZA DOUGH	161	.5	3
SPICY SPANISH OMELETTE	102	.5	4
OVEN STEAMED RED BLISS POTATOES	273	.5	2
HONEYDEW HONEY	212	.5	2
VEGETABLE STOCK	41	.6	11
QUICK FRUIT AND FIBER SNACK	25	.6	20
CHAMPAGNE BALSAMIC VINAIGRETTE	24	.6	47
GRILLED SEAFOOD SAUSAGE	83	.7	8
CHILLED FRUIT SOUP	129	.8	5
APPLE FRAPPE	287	1.0	3
ROASTED GARLIC AND NORTHERN BEAN SPREAD	55	1.0	16
MARINATED NORTHERN AND TURTLE BEANS	343	1.1	3
CREAM SAUCE	41	1.2	24
BREAKFAST #1	283	1.2	4
SAUTEED PINEAPPLE WITH STRAWBERRY YOGURT SAUCE	256	1.2	4
BLACK BEAN SAUCE OR DIP	159	1.3	9
HEARTY FIVE BEAN SOUP	245	1.3	5
POACHED BARTLETT PEAR AND KIWI BRANDY SAUCE	236	1.3	5

RECIPE	CAL	FAT GM	FAT %
BREAKFAST #5	469	1.4	3
VEGETABLE KABOBS	155	1.4	8
SPICY NAPA COLE SLAW	61	1.4	18
MARINATED ASPARAGUS SPEARS	106	1.5	11
CHARBROILED BEEFSTEAK TOMATO SALAD	97	1.5	11
OVEN POACHED SCROD AND WILD GREENS	208	1.5	6
DRIED CHERRY AND ORANGE COOKIES	70	1.5	19
HERBED RICE PILAF	141	1.6	10
CHEESE BLINTZES	129	1.6	11
CASCADE COLADA	328	1.8	5
VEGETABLE CHILI	131	1.9	12
CHICKEN SATAY APPETIZER	92	1.9	18
YOGURT CUCUMBER DILL SAUCE	30	1.9	56
SEAFOOD RAVIOLI	338	2.0	5
GEORGIA PEACH BEGGARS PURSE	196	2.0	9
FARFELLA WITH SWEET BASIL AND LENTILS	359	2.1	5
THE DELMONTE	229	2.2	6
OVEN ROASTED VEGETABLE MARINARA SAUCE	71	2.3	25
GINGER LIME VINAIGRETTE	26	2.3	74
RATAOUILLIE	98	2.4	19
RED BEANS AND RICE	246	2.4	9
BASIC CHICKEN STOCK	49	2.4	41
BREAKFAST #3	544	2.5	4
TURKEY MEATLOAF	220	2.6	11
STUFFED CHICKEN BREAST NORTHCOAST WITH TOMATO BASIL SAUCE	248	2.6	9
RED WINE HERB MARINADE	90	2.6	39
APPLE COBBLER	214	2.6	11
BRAISED FENNEL	99	2.7	22
OVEN FRIED CHICKEN BREAST	218	2.8	12
QUICK ORIENTAL EGG DROP SOUP	73	2.8	34
POACHED STUFFED BONELESS BREAST OF CHICKEN	285	3.1	10

RECIPE	CAL	FAT GM	FAT %
MAPLE WALNUT RAISIN MUFFINS	175	3.1	15
TWICE BAKED POTATO	146	3.3	19
RAINBOW ROTINI WITH CHARBROILED VEGETABLES	684	3.8	5
GRILLED SHRIMP AND WARM VEGETABLE SALAD CAPELLINI	577	4.0	6
EGGPLANT PARMESAN	266	4.2	13
BREAKFAST #7	632	4.2	6
CHOCOLATE MINT CAROB PUDDING	246	4.2	14
TUNA STUFFED BEEFSTEAK TOMATO	440	4.5	8
GRILLED VEGETARIAN SANDWICH WITH WHOLE WHEAT PITA BREAD	322	4.6	11
BANANA PEPPERS AND SPINACH SALAD	185	4.7	19
CASHEW CRUSTED ORANGE ROUGHY	131	4.8	31
BERRY BANANA DELIGHT	537	5.0	7
STRAWBERRY YOGURT SMOOTHIE	473	5.0	8
PEPPER STEAK BARLEY SOUP	193	5.3	23
CHARBROILED BONELESS BREAST OF CHICKEN WITH PINEAPPLE CHUTNEY	300	5.5	16
SHRIMP AND BARLEY SALAD	900	5.6	5
THE BRAZIEL	358	5.7	14
PIZZA SAUCE	142	5.8	32
GINGERED CASHEW CHICKEN	500	6.2	11
GRILLED SEA SCALLOPS AND WAX BEANS	199	6.4	25
GRILLED SESAME HALIBUT AND LEAF SPINACH SALAD	236	6.5	23
CHARBROILED HALIBUT STEAKS WITH CILANTRO CITRUS SAUCE	686	6.9	9
POACHED ATLANTIC SALMON FILLET	495	7.1	12
GRILLED SWORDFISH STEAK	413	7.1	15
JULIENNE VEGETABLE CHOW MEIN	578	7.5	11
BREAKFAST #6	450	8.0	16
CASABLANCA TURKEY SALAD	281	8.0	26
GERMAN TOMATO AND CUCUMBER SALAD	283	8.0	23
BREAKFAST #4	290	8.1	23

RECIPE	CAL	FAT GM	FAT %
CREOLE CATFISH	272	8.1	29
GRILLED BREAST OF CHICKEN PALOMBO	257	8.3	28
CHICKEN AND ARTICHOKE SALAD	485	8.7	15
CHICKEN WALDORF SALAD	618	9.0	12
SPINACH AND BEAN ENCHILADAS	368	9.4	22
SPAGHETTI CARBONARA	586	9.7	15
POLENTA, MUSHROOMS AND MARINARA SAUCE	364	10.0	24
PESTO SAUCE	107	10.0	80
GRILLED SESAME HALIBUT AND LEAF SPINACH SALAD	325	10.3	28
TOMATO FETTUCCINE WITH MARINARA SAUCE AND ZUCCHINI	614	10.4	15
CHICKEN ALMOND STIR FRY	318	11.2	31
BARLEY AND PECAN BREAST OF CHICKEN	368	11.5	28
BREAKFAST #8	599	11.6	17
GROUND TURKEY BURGER	468	11.6	22
BREAKFAST #2	649	12.2	16
LINGUINI, HAM AND GREEN PEAS	569	12.2	19
TURKEY PARMESAN	436	12.8	26
PENNA PASTA AND JULIENNE VEGETABLES	1134	13.2	10
HERB BAKED CANADIAN PICKEREL	419	14.6	30
COUSCOUS & GRILLED ONION HAMBURGER	398	16.1	35
HAMBURGER WITH PEARLED BARLEY	492	16.7	29
REDUCED FAT HAMBURGER	487	17.0	30
GRILLED TENDERLOIN OF BEEF AND COUSCOUS SALAD	662	17.9	24
STADIUM PEARLBURGER	566	18.3	28
COURT BOUILLON USED FOR POACHING SEAFOOD	1297	19.1	12
ANGEL HAIR WITH PESTO AND GRILLED EGGPLANT	680	20.0	26
NORTH CAROLINA GRILLED TROUT	848	22.5	25
BEEF MEDALLIONS AND JICAMA	1001	23.0	22
PORK TENDERLOIN WITH ZITA SALAD	848	23.0	24

FOOTNOTES

1. Daily dietary fat and total food-energy-intakes, Third National Health and Nutrition Examination Survey, Phase 1, 1988-1991, MMWR - Morbidity & Mortality Weekly Report, 43(7):116-7, 123-5, 1994 Feb. 25.
2. Lissner, L., Department of Medicine, University of Goteborg, Sweden, Adipose tissue fatty acids and dietary fat sources in relation to endometrial cancer: a retrospective study of cases in remission, and population-based controls, Acta Obstetricia et Gynecologica Scandinavica, 72(6):481-7, 1993 Aug.
3. Weisburger, J., Jones, R., American Health Foundation, Valhalla, New York, Prevention of formation of important mutagens/carcinogens in the human food chain, [Review] Basic Life Sciences, 52:105-18, 1990.
4. Roebuck, B., Department of Pharmacology and Toxicology, Dartmouth Medical School, Hanover, New Hampshire, Dietary fat and the development of pancreatic cancer, [Review] Lipids, 27(10):804-6, 1992 Oct.
5. Freudenheim, J., Graham, S., Department of Social and Preventive Medicine, State University of New York, Buffalo, Diet, smoking, and alcohol in cancer of the larynx: a case-control study, Nutrition and Cancer, 17(1):33-45, 1992.
6. Hirayama, T., Institute of Preventive Oncology, Tokyo, Japan, Life-style and cancer: from epidemiological evidence to public behavior change to mortality reduction of target cancers, Monographs - National Cancer Institute, (12):65-74, 1992.
7. Graham, S., Department of Social and Preventive Medicine, State University of New York, Diet in the epidemiology of postmenopausal breast cancer in the New York State Cohort, American Journal of Epidemiology, 136(11):1327-37, 1992 Dec 1.
8. Ziegler, R., Vegetables, fruits, and carotenoids and the risk of cancer, Am J of Clinical Nutri, 53 (1 Suppl):251S-259S, 1991 Jan.
9. Decosse, J., et al., Effect of wheat fiber and vitamins C and E on rectal polyps in patients with familial adenomatous polyosis, J Nat'l Cancer Instit, 81(17):1290-7, 1989 Sep 6.
10. Van't Veer, P., et al., Combination of dietary factors in relation to breast cancer occurrence, Internat'l J Cancer, 47(5):649-53, 1991 Mar. 12.
11. Howe, G., et al., A collaborative case-control study of nutrient intake and pancreatic cancer within the search programme, Internat'l J Cancer, 51(3):365-72, 1992 May 28.
12. Van't Veer, P., et al., Dietary fiber, beta-carotene and breast cancer: results from a case-control study, Internat'l J Cancer, 45(5):825-8, 1990 May 15.
13. Gallaher, D., et al., Bile acid metabolism in rats fed two levels of corn oil and brans of oat, rye and barley and sugar beet fiber, J Nutri, 122(3):473-81, 1992 Mar.
14. Rohan, R., et al., Dietary fiber, vitamin A, C, and E, and risk of breast cancer: a cohort study, Cancer Causes & Control, 4(1):29-37, 1993 Jan.
15. Zaridze, D., et al., Diet and colorectal cancer: results of two case-control studies in Russia, European J Cancer, 29A(1):112-5, 1992.
16. Mettlin, C., et al., Beta-carotene and animal fats and their relationship to prostate cancer risk, a case-control study, Cancer, 64(3):605-12, 1989 Aug. 1.
17. Corcos, Benedetti, et al., Influence of dietary thermally oxidized soybean oil on the oxidative status of rats of different ages, Ans Nutri & Metabol, 34(4):221-31, 1990.
18. Negri, E., et al., Attributable risks for oesophageal cancer in northern Italy, European J Cancer, 28A(6-7):1167-71, 1992.

19. Nishikawa, A., et al., Effects of caffeine, nicotine, ethanol and sodium selenite on pancreatic carcinogenesis in hamsters after initiation with N-nitrosobis (2-oxopropyl)amine, Carcinogenesis, 13(8):1379-82, 1992 Aug.

20. Stryker, W., et al., Diet, plasma levels of beta-carotene and alpha-tocopherol, and risk of malignant melanoma, Am J Epidemiol, 131(4):597-611, 1990 Apr.

21. Lee, D., et al., Modulation of free radicals and superoxide dismutases by age and dietary restriction, Aging, 2(4):357-62, 1990 Dec.

22. Ishigami, A., et al., Effect of dietary restriction on the degradation of proteins in senescent mouse liver parenchymal cells in culture, Arch of Biochem & Biophys, 283(2):362-6, 1990 Dec.

23. Mote, P., et al., Influence of age and caloric restriction on expression of hepatic genes for xenobiotic and oxygen metabolizing enzymes in the mouse, J Gerontol, 46(3):B95-100, 1992 May.

24. Rao, G., et al., Effect of dietary restriction and the age-dependent changes in the expression of antioxidant enzymes in rat liver, J Nutri, 120(6):602-9, 1990 Jun.

25. Laganiere, S., et al., Effect of chronic food restriction in aging rats, II, Liver cytosolic antioxidants and related enzymes, Mech of Aging & Develop, 48(3):221-30, 1989 Jun.

26. Bonkovsky, H., Iron and the liver, Amer J Med Sci, 301(1):32-43, 1991 Jan.

27. Weisburger, J.H., American Health Foundation, Valhalla, New York, Dietary fat intake and cancer, [Review] Hematology - Oncology Clinics of North America, 5(1):7-23, 1991 Feb.

28. Vatten, L.J., Institutt for miljo- og, samfunnsmedisinske fag, Medisinsk Teknisk Senter, Trondheim, [Diet and cancer risk], [Norwegian] Original Title Kosthold og kreftrisiko, Tidsskrift for Den Norske Laegeforening, 114(6):702-5, 1994 Feb 28.

29. Byers, T., Center for Disease Control and Prevention, National Center for Chronic Disease Prevention and Health Promotion, Atlanta, Georgia 30341-3724, Dietary trends in the United States, Relevance to cancer prevention, [Review] Cancer, 72(3 Suppl):1015-8, 1993 Aug 1.

30. Prentice, R.L., Sheppard L. Division of Public Health Sciences, Fred Hutchinson Cancer Research Center, Seattle WA 98104, Dietary fat and cancer: consistency of the epidemiologic data, and disease prevention that may follow from a practical reduction in fat consumption [published erratum appears in Cancer Causes Control 1990 Nov;1(3):253], [Review] Cancer Causes & Control, 1(1):81-97; discussion 99-109, 1990 Jul.

31. Birt, D.F., Eppley Institute for Research in Cancer, University of Nebraska Medical Center, Omaha 68105, The influence of dietary fat on carcinogenesis: lessons from experimental models, [Review] Nutrition Reviews, 48(1):1-5, 1990 Jan.

32. Rolls, B.J., Shide, D.J., College of Health and Human Development, Pennsylvania State University, University Park 16802-6508, The influence of dietary fat on food intake and body weight [published erratum appears in Nutr Rev 1993 Jan;51(1):31], [Review] Nutrition Reviews, 50(10):283-90, 1992 Oct.

33. Ling, P.R., Istfan NW, Cancer Research Institute, New England Deaconess Hospital, Boston, MA 02215, Structured lipid made from fish oil and medium-chain triglycerides alters tumor and host metabolism in Yoshida-sarcoma-bearing rats, American Journal of Clinical Nutrition 53(5):177-84, 1991 May.

34. Mizukami, Y., Nonomura, A., Pathology Section, Kanazawa University Hospital, Japan, Effects of high and low dietary fat and indomethacin on tumour growth, hormone receptor status and growth factor expression in DMBA-induced rat breast cancer, International Journal of Tissue Reactions, 14(6):269-76, 1992.

35. Holm, L.E., Department of Cancer Prevention, Radiumhemmet, Karolinska Hospital, Stockholm, Sweden, Dietary intervention as adjuvant therapy in breast cancer patients—a feasibility study, Breast Cancer Research & Treatment, 16(2):103-9, 1990 Sep.

36. Greenwald, P., Division of Cancer Prevention and Control, National Cancer Institute, National Institutes of Health, Bethesda, MD 20892, Keynote address: cancer prevention, Monographs -National Cancer Institute, (12):9-14, 1992.

37. Gonzalez, M.J., Rodriguez, J.R., Michigan State University, East Lansing 48823, Fat and breast cancer: a mini-review of experimental data on rodents, Boletin - Asociacion Medica de Puerto Rico, 83(6):264-6, 1991 Jun.

38. Rose, D.P., Connolly, J.M., Division of Nutrition and Endocrinology, American Health Foundation, Valhalla, NY 10595, Influence of dietary fat intake on local recurrence and progression of metastases arising from MDA-MB-435 human breast cancer cells in nude mice after excision of the primary tumor, Nutrition & Cancer, 18(2):113-22, 1992.

39. Rose, D.P., Connolly, J.M., Division of Nutrition and Endocrinology, American Health

Foundation, Valhalla, New York, Dietary prevention of breast cancer, [Review] Medical Oncology & Tumor Pharmacotherapy, 7(2-3):121-30, 1990.

40. Hankin, J.H., Epidemiology Program, Cancer Research Center of Hawaii, University of Hawaii, Honolulu 96813, Role of nutrition in women's health: diet and breast cancer [see comments], [Review] Journal of the American Dietetic Association, 93(9):994-9, 1993 Sep.

41. Morabia, A., Wynder, E.L., Division of Epidemiology, Columbia University School of Public Health, New York, New York, Epidemiology and natural history of breast cancer, Implications for the body weight-breast cancer controversy, [Review] Surgical Clinics of North America, 70(4):739-52, 1990 Aug.

42. Barrett-Connor, E., Friedlander, N.J., Dept. of Family and Preventive Medicine, University of California, San Diego, La Jolla 92093-0607, Dietary fat, calories, and the risk of breast cancer in postmenopausal women: a prospective population-based study, Journal of the American College of Nutrition, 12(4):390-9, 1993 Aug.

43. Rose, D.P., Division of Nutrition and Endocrinology, American Health Foundation, Valhalla, New York, Dietary fiber, phytoestrogens, and breast cancer, [Review] Nutrition, 8(1):47-51, 1992 Jan-Feb.

44. Boyd, N.F., McGuire, V., Department of Medicine, Ontario Cancer Institute, Toronto, Canada, Evidence of association between plasma high-density lipoprotein cholesterol and risk factors for breast cancer, Journal of the National Cancer Institute, 82(6):460-8, 1990 Mar 21.

45. Sasaki, S., Horacsek, M., Kesteloot H, Department of Epidemiology, School of Public Health, University of Leuven, Belgium, An ecological study of the relationship between dietary fat intake and breast cancer mortality, Preventive Medicine, 22(2):187-202, 1993 Mar.

46. Howe, G.R., Friedenreich CM, National Cancer Institute of Canada Epidemiology Unit, Faculty of Medicine, University of Toronto, ON, A cohort study of fat intake and risk of breast cancer [see comments], Journal of the National Cancer Institute, 83(5):336-40, 1991 Mar 6.

47. Richardson, S., Inserm U.170, Montpellier, France, The role of fat, animal protein and some vitamin consumption in breast cancer: a case control study in southern France, International Journal of Cancer, 48(1):1-9, 1991 Apr 22.

48. Furst, C.J., Department of General Oncology, Karolinska Hospital, Stockholm, Sweden, DNA pattern and dietary habits in patients with breast cancer, European Journal of Cancer, 29A(9):1285-8, 1993.

49. Holm, L.E., Nordevang E, Department of Cancer Prevention, Radiumhemmet, Karolinska Hospital, Stockholm, Sweden, Treatment failure and dietary habits in women with breast cancer, Journal of the National Cancer Institute, 85(1):32-6, 1993 Jan 6.

50. Van't Veer, P., Kok, F.J., TNO-CIVO Toxicology and Nutrition Institute, Zeist, The Netherlands, Dietary fat and the risk of breast cancer, International Journal of Epidemiology, 19(1):12-8, 1990 Mar.

51. Knekt, P., Research Institute for Social Security, Social Insurance Institution, Helsinki, Finland, Dietary fat and risk of breast cancer, American Journal of Clinical Nutrition, 52 (5):903-8, 1990 Nov.

52. Salim, A.S., University Department of Surgery, Royal Infirmary, Glasgow, UK, The permissive role of oxygen-derived free radicals in the development of colonic cancer in the rat, A new theory for carcinogenesis, International Journal of Cancer, 53(6):1031-5, 1993 Apr 1.

53. Steinbach, G., Department of Medicine, St. Luke's/Roosevelt Hospital Center, New York, Effects of caloric restriction and dietary fat on epithelial cell proliferation in rat colon, Cancer Research, 53(12):2745-9, 1993 Jun 15.

54. Burnstein, M.J., Department of Surgery, University of Toronto, Ontario, Canada, Dietary factors related to colorectal neoplasms, [Review] Surgical Clinics of North America, 73(1):13-29, 1993 Feb.

55. Gallaher, D.D., Locket, P.L., Gallaher, C.M., Department of Food Science and Nutrition, University of Minnesota, St. Paul 55108, Bile acid metabolism in rats fed two levels of corn oil and brans of oat, rye and barley and sugar beet fiber, Journal of Nutrition, 122(3):473-81, 1992 Mar.

56. Thun, M.J., Calle, E.E., Epidemiology Division, Emory University School of Public Health, Atlanta, Ga, Risk factors for fatal colon cancer in a large prospective study [see comments], Journal of the National Cancer Institute, 84(19):1491-500, 1992 Oct 7.

57. Graham, S., Department of Social and Preventive Medicine, State University of New York

14214, Diet in the epidemiology of postmenopausal breast cancer in the New York State Cohort, American Journal of Epidemiology, 136(11):1327-37, 1992 Dec 1.

58. Statland, B.E., National Reference Laboratory, Nashville, TN 37217, Nutrition and cancer, [Review] Clinical Chemistry, 38(8B Pt 2):1587-94, 1992 Aug.

59. Miller, A.B., Department of Preventive Medicine and Biostatistics, University of Toronto, Ontario, Canada, Diet and cancer, A review, [Review] Acta Oncologica, 29(1):87-95, 1990.

60. Carroll, K.K., Department of Biochemistry, University of Western Ontario, London, Canada, Dietary fats and cancer, [Review] American Journal of Clinical Nutrition. 53(4 Suppl):1064S-1067S, 1991 Apr.

61. Yu, H., Harris, R.E., American Health Foundation, New York 10017, Comparative epidemiology of cancers of the colon, rectum, prostate and breast in Shanghai, China versus the United States, International Journal of Epidemiology, 20(1):76-81, 1991 Mar.

62. Weisburger, J.H., American Health Foundation, Valhalla, New York, Dietary fat intake and cancer, [Review] Hematology-Oncology Clinics of North America, 5(1):7-23, 1991 Feb.

63. Browner, W.S., Westenhouse, J., Department of Medicine, Veterans Affairs Medical Center, San Francisco, CA 94121, What if Americans ate less fat?, A quantitative estimate of the effect on mortality [see comments], JAMA, 265(24):3285-91, 1991 Jun 26.

64. Miller, A.B., Epidemiological approaches to primary and secondary prevention of cancer [editorial], Journal of Cancer Research & Clinical Oncology, 117(3):177-85, 1991.

65. Henderson, M.M., Division of Public Health Sciences, Fred Hutchinson Cancer Research Center, Seattle, WA 98104, International differences in diet and cancer incidence, Monographs - National Cancer Institute, (12):59-63, 1992.

66. Hirayama, T., Institute of Preventive Oncology, Tokyo, Japan, Life-style and cancer: from epidemiological evidence to public behavior change to mortality reduction of target cancers, Monographs - National Cancer Institute, (12):65-74, 1992.

67. Hursting, S.D., Thornquist, M., Henderson, M.M., Cancer Prevention Research Program, Fred Hutchinson Cancer Research Center, Seattle, Washington 98104, Types of dietary fat and the incidence of cancer at five sites, Preventive Medicine, 19(3):242-53, 1990 May.

68. Browner, W.S., Westenhouse, J., Department of Medicine, Veterans Affairs Medical Center, San Francisco, CA 94121, What if Americans ate less fat?, A quantitative estimate of the effect on mortality [see comments], JAMA, 265(24):3285-91, 1991 Jun 26.

69. Pienta, K.J., Meyer, L., Prentis Comprehensive Cancer Center of Metropolitan Detroit, Michigan, Risk factors for prostate cancer, [Review] Annals of Internal Medicine, 118(10):793-803, 1993 May 15.

70. Giovannucci, E., Rimm, E.B., Channing Laboratory, Department of Medicine, Harvard Medical School, Boston, Mass, A prospective study of dietary fat and risk of prostate cancer [see comments], Journal of the National Cancer Institute, 85(19):1571-9, 1993 Oct 6.

71. Statland, B.E., National Reference Laboratory, Nashville, TN 37217, Nutrition and cancer, [Review] Clinical Chemistry, 38(8B Pt 2):1587-94, 1992 Aug.

72. Yu, H., Harris, R.E., American Health Foundation, New York 10017, Comparative epidemiology of cancers of the colon, rectum, prostate and breast in Shanghai, China versus the United States, International Journal of Epidemiology, 20(1):76-81, 1991 Mar.

73. Hursting, S.D., Thornquist, M., Henderson, M.M., Cancer Prevention Research Program, Fred Hutchinson Cancer Research Center, Seattle, Washington 98104, Types of dietary fat and the incidence of cancer at five sites, Preventive Medicine, 19(3):242-53, 1990 May.

74. West, D.W., Northern California Cancer Center, Adult dietary intake and prostate cancer risk in Utah: a case-control study with special emphasis on aggressive tumors, Cancer Causes & Control, 2(2):85-94, 1991 Mar.

75. Meikle, A.W., Smith, J.A. Jr., Department of Medicine, University of Utah Center for the Health Sciences, Salt Lake City, Epidemiology of prostate cancer, [Review] Urologic Clinics of North America, 17(4):709-18, 1990 Nov.

76. Anderson, R., Assessment of the roles of vitamin C, vitamin E, and beta-carotene in the modulation of oxidant stress mediated by cigarette smoke-activated phagocytes, Am J Clinical Nutri, 53(1 Suppl):358s-361s, 1991 Jan.

77. Singh, V., et al., Premalignant lesions: role of antioxidant vitamins and beta-carotene in risk reduction and prevention of malignant transformation, Am J Clinical Nutri, 53(1 Suppl):386S-390S, 1991 Jan.

78. Palan, P., et al., Plasma levels of antioxidant beta-carotene and alpha-tocopherol in uter-

ine cervix dysplasias and cancer, 15(1):13-20, 1991

79. Nagasawa, H., et al., Suppression by beta-carotene-rich algae dunaliella bardawil of the progression, but not the development, of spontaneous mammary tumours in shn virgin Mice, Anticancer Res, 11(2):713-7, 1991 Mar-Apr.

80. Bianchi, L., et al., Reduction of chromosomal damage by bleomycin in lymphocytes from subjects supplemented with carotenoids. relevance in bleomycin tumour chemotherapy. Preliminary results, Bollet Chim Farmaceutico, 129(12):83S-87S, 1990 Dec.

81. Zaman, Z., et al., Plasma concentrations of vitamins A and E and carotenoids in Alzheimer's disease, Age & Ageing, 21(2):91-4, 1992 Mar.

82. Toma, S., et al., In vitro effects of beta-carotene on human oral keratinocytes from pre-cancerous lesion and squamous carcinoma, Anti-Cancer Drugs, 2(6):581-9, 1991 Dec.

83. Eichholzer, M., et al., Inverse correlation between essential antioxidants in plasma and subsequent risk to develop cancer, ischemic heart disease and stroke respectively: 12-year follow-up of the prospective Basel study, EXS, 62:398-410, 1992.

84. Nagasawa, H., et al., Suppression by beta-carotene-rich algae dunaliella bardawil of the progression, but not the development, of spontaneous mammary tumours in shn virgin mice, Anticancer Res, 11(2):713-7, 1991 Mar-Apr.

85. Maleskey, Gale, A Doctor's Guide to Anti-Aging Nutrients Prevention, (Pennsylvania, Rodale Press), 1985.

86. From the American Cancer Society, National Research Council, and the National Cancer Institute.

87. Diet, Nutrition and Cancer, Washington National Academy Press, 1992.

88. Stahelin, H., Vitamins and cancer: results of a Basel study, 34(2):75-7, 1989.

89. Eichholzer, M., et al., Inverse correlation between essential antioxidants in plasma and subsequent risk to develop cancer, ischemic heart disease and stroke respectively: 12-year follow-up of the prospective Basel study, EXS, 62:398-410, 1992.

90. Abril, E., et al., Beta-carotene stimulates human leukocytes to secrete a novel cytokine, J Leukocyte Biol, 45(3):255-61, 1986 Mar.

91. Connett, J., et al., Relationship between carotenoids and cancer, The multiple risk factor intervention trial (MRFIT) study, Internat'l J Dev Neurosci, 64(1):126-34, 1989 Jul 1.

92. Slattery, M., et al., Nutrient intake and ovarian cancer, Ans Cardiol et Angeilolgie, 130(3):497-502, 1989 Sep.

93. Schwartz, J., et al., Induction of a 70 KD protein associated with the selective cytotoxicity of beta-carotene in human epidermal carcinoma, Biochem & Biol Res Comm, 169(3):941-6, 1990 Jun 29.

94. Schwartz, J., et al., The selective cytotoxic effect of carotenoids and alpha-tocopherol on human cancer cell lines in vitro, J Oral & Maxillofacial Surg, 50(4):367-73; Disc. 373-4, 1992 Apr.

95. Bendich, Adrianne, Carotenoids and the Immune Response, J Nutri, 119:112-115, 1989.

96. Smith, A., et al., Serum beta-carotene in persons with cancer and their immediate families, Am J Epidemiol, 133(7):661-71, 1991 Apr 1.

97. Li, Y., et al., Correlation of selenium, glutathione peroxidase activity and lipoperoxidation rates in dilated cardiomyopathy, Chin Med J - Peking, 102(9):670-1, 1989 Sep.

98. Kise, Y., et al., Inhibitory effect of selenium on hamster pancreatic cancer induction by N-nitrosobis (2-oxopropylamine, Internat'l J Cancer, 46(1):95-100, 1990 Jul 15.

99. Yan, L., et al., Effect of selenium compounds and thiols on human mammary tumor cells, Biol Trace Element Res, 30(2):145-62, 1991 Aug.

100. Pawlowicz, Z., et al., Blood selenium concentrations and glutathione peroxidase activities in patients with breast cancer and with advanced gastrointestinal cancer, J Trace Elem & Electrolytes, 5(4):275-7, 1991 Dec.

101. Selvam, R., et al., Restoration of antioxidants in liver by methionine feeding in experimental rat urolithiasis, Ind J Biochem & Biophysics, 29(4):364-70, 1992 Aug.

102. Kumar, K., et al., Changes observed in antioxidant system in the blood of post-menopausal women with breast cancer, Biochem Internat'l, 25(2):371-80, 1991 Sep.

103. Kumar, K., et al., Changes observed in antioxidant system in the blood of post-menopausal women with breast cancer, Biochem Internat'l, 25(2):371-80, 1991 Sep.

104. Crastes Depaulet, Free radicals and aging, Ans Biologie Clinique, 48(5):323-30, 1990

105. Kuvshinnikov, V., et al., Use of the antioxidant complex of vitamins A, E and C in murine leukemia, Gematologiia/Transfuziologiia, 34(8):23-8, 1989 Aug.

106. Balabolkin, I., et al., Use of vitamins in allergic illnesses in children, Voprosy Meditsinskoi Khimii, 38(5):36-40, 1992 Sep.-Oct.

107. Negre-Salvayre, et al., Quercetin prevents the cytotoxicity of oxidized LDL on lymphoid

cell lines, Free Rad Biol & Med, 12(2):101-6, 1992

108. Reznick, A., et al., The threshold of age in exercise and antioxidants action, EXS, 62:423-7, 1992.

109. El Attar, T., et al., Effect of vitamin C and vitamin E on prostaglandin synthesis by fibroblasts and squamous carcinoma cells, Prostagland Leukot & Essen FA, 47(4):253-7, 1992 Dec.

110. Stahelin, H., et al., Plasma antioxidant vitamins and subsequent cancer mortality in the 12-year follow-up of the prospective Basel study, Am J Epidemiol, 133(8):766-75, 1991 Apr 15.

111. Jaskiewicz, K., et al., Chronic atrophic gastritis, gastric PH, nitrites and micronutrient levels in a population at risk for gastric carcinoma, Anticancer Res, 10(3):833-6, 1990 May-Jun.

112. Cameron, E., et al., Innovation vs. quality control: an unpublishable clinical trial of supplemental ascorbate in incurable cancer, Med Hypotheses, 36(3):185-9, 1991 Nov.

113. Nitta, Y., et al., Induction of transplantable tumors by repeated subcutaneous injections of natural and synthetic vitamin E in mice and rats, Jap J Cancer Res, 82(5):511-7, 1991 May.

114. Corcos, Benedetti, et al., Influence of dietary thermally oxidized soybean oil on the oxidative status of rats of different ages, Ans Nutri & Metabol, 34(4):221-31, 1990.

115. Alexander, J., et al., Future prospects for adjunctive therapy: pharmacologic and nutritional approaches to immune system modulation, Critical Care Med, 18(2 Suppl):s159-64, 1990 Feb.

116. Knekt, P., et al., Vitamin E and cancer prevention, Am J Clinical Nutri, 53(1 Suppl):283S-286S, 1991 Jan.

117. He, R., Inhibitory effect of micronutrients and BHA on lung cancer induced in rats, Chung-hau Chung Liu Tsa Chih, 12(6):421-4, 1990 Nov.

118. Rao, A., et al., Modulatory influences of tamoxifen, tocopherol, retinyl acetate, aminoglutethimide, ergocryptine and selenium on dmba-induced initiation of mammary carcinogenesis in rats, Indian J Exper Biol, 28(5):409-16, 1990 May.

119. Kuvshinnikov, V., et al., Use of the antioxidant complex of vitamins A, E and C in murine leukemia, Gematologiia/Transfuziologiia, 34(8):23-8, 1989 Aug.

120. Thompson, H., Effect of deficiencies of selenium and vitamin E alone or in combination on the induction of mammary carcinogenesis by 1-methyl-1-nitro sources, Carcinogenesis, 12(11):2175-9, 1991 Nov.

121. El Attar, T., et al., Effect of vitamin C and vitamin E on crostaglandin synthesis by fibroblasts and squamous carcinoma cells, Prostagland Leukot & Essen FA, 47(4):253-7, 1992 Dec.

122. Shklar, G., et al., Prevention of experimental cancer and immunostimulation by vitamin E (immunosurveillance), J Oral Pathol & Med, 19(2):60-4, 1990 Feb.

123. Colacchio, T., et al., Antioxidants vs carotenoids. Inhibitors or promotes of experimental colorectal cancers, Arch of Surg, 124(2):217-21, 1989 Feb.

124. Kishino, Y., et al., Nutritional factors and cellular immune responses, Nutrition & Health, 8(2-3):133-41, 1992.

125. Leibovitz, B., et al., Dietary supplements of vitamin E, beta-carotene, coenzyme Q10 and selenium protect tissues against lipid peroxidation in rat tissue slices, J Nutri, 120(1):97-104, 1990 Jan.

126. Soderberg, M., et al., Lipid compositions of different regions of the human brain during aging, J Neuochem, 54(2):415-23, 1990 Feb.

127. Edlund, C., et al., Ubiquinone, dolichol, and cholesterol metabolism in aging and Alzheimer's disease, Biochem & Cell Biol, 70(6):422-8, 1992 Jun.

128. Kalen, A., et al., Age-related changes in the lipid compositions of rat and human tissues, Lipids, 24(7):579-84, 1989 Jul.

129. Vitullo, F., Di Mascio, R., Istituto di Ricerche Farmacologiche Mario Negri Laboratorio di Farmacologia Clinica ed Epidemiologia, Consorzio Mario Negri Sud S, Maria Imbaro, Chieti, [Can the changes in dietary fat intake reduce the risk of onset and development of atherosclerosis and of ischemic cardiopathy in particular?], [Italian] Original Title Puo la modificazione dei grassi alimentari ridurre il rischio di insorgenza e sviluppo dell'aterosclerosi ed in particolare della cardiopatia ischemica? Giornale Italiano di Cardiologia, 21(4):361-74, 1991 Apr.

130. Browner, W.S., Westenhouse, J., Department of Medicine, Veterans Affairs Medical Center, San Francisco, CA 94121, What if Americans ate less fat?, A quantitative estimate of the effect on mortality [see comments], JAMA, 265(24):3285-91, 1991 Jun 26.

131. Rolls, B.J., Shide, D.J., College of Health and Human Development, Pennsylvania State University, University Park 16802-6508, The influence of dietary fat on food intake and body weight [published erratum appears in Nutr Rev 1993 Jan;51(1):31], [Review] Nutrition Reviews, 50(10):283-90, 1992 Oct.

132. Cunnane, S.C., Department of Nutritional Sciences, Faculty of Medicine, University of Toronto, Canada, Childhood origins of lifestyle-related risk factors for coronary heart disease in adulthood, [Review] Nutrition & Health, 9(2):107-15, 1993.

133. Connor, W.E., Connor, S.L., Department of Medicine, Oregon Health Sciences University, Portland 97201-3098, Importance of diet in the treatment of familial hypercholesterolemia, [Review] American Journal of Cardiology, 72(10):42D-53D, 1993 Sep 30.

134. Sharlin, J., Posner, B.M., Department of Health Sciences, Boston University, Mass, Nutrition and behavioral characteristics and determinants of plasma cholesterol levels in men and women, Journal of the American Dietetic Association, 92(4):434-40, 1992 Apr.

135. Ninomiya, K., Maruhama, Y., 1st Department of Internal Medicine, Iwate Medical University, School of Medicine, Morioka, [Borderline values of laboratory data in patients with hyperlipidemia], [Japanese] Rinsho Byori - Japanese Journal of Clinical Pathology, 41(6):627-31, 1993 Jun.

136. Wolfe, M.S., Parks, J.S., Department of Biochemistry, Bowman Gray School of Medicine, Wake Forest University, Winston-Salem, N.C. 27157-1040, Childhood consumption of dietary polyunsaturated fat lowers risk for coronary artery atherosclerosis in African green monkeys, Arteriosclerosis & Thrombosis, 13(6):863-75, 1993 Jun.

137. Haskell, W.L., Alderman, E.L., Division of Cardiovascular Medicine, Stanford University, Palo Alto, CA 94304-1583, Effects of intensive multiple risk factor reduction on coronary atherosclerosis and clinical cardiac events in men and women with coronary artery disease, The Stanford Coronary Risk Intervention Project (SCRIP), Circulation 89(3):975-90, 1994 Mar.

138. Connor, W.E., Connor, S.L., Department of Medicine, Oregon Health Sciences University, Portland, Diet, atherosclerosis, and fish oil, [Review] Advances in Internal Medicine, 35:139-71, 1990.

139. Iacono, J.M., Dougherty, R.M., USDA-ARS, Western Human Nutrition Research Center, Presidio of San Francisco, California, Dietary fat and blood pressure in humans, [Review] Klinische Wochenschrift, 68 Suppl 20:23-32, 1990.

140. Sabate, J., Fraser, G.E., Center for Health Research, School of Public Health, Loma Linda University, CA 92350, Effects of walnuts on serum lipid levels and blood pressure in normal men [see comments], New England Journal of Medicine, 328(9):603-7, 1993 Mar 4.

141. Stein, P.P., Black, H.R., Department of Internal Medicine, Yale University School of Medicine, Hew Haven, Connecticut, The role of diet in the genesis and treatment of hypertension, Medical Clinics of North America, 77(4):831-47, 1993 Jul.

142. Stephen, A.M., Wald, N.J., Division of Nutrition and Dietetics, College of Pharmacy, University of Saskatchewan Saskatton, Canada, Trends in individual consumption of dietary fat in the United States, 1920-1984, American Journal of Clinical Nutrition, 52(3):457-69, 1990 Sep.

143. Heikkila, M., [The role of dietary fats in health], [Finnish] Original Title Rasvan laadulla on merkitysta, Sairaanhoitaja Sjukskoterskan, (7):19-20, 1993.

144. Tzonou, A., Kalandidi, A., Department of Hygiene and Epidemiology, University of Athens Medical School, Greece, Diet and coronary heart disease: a case-control study in Athens, Greece [see comments], Epidemiology, 4(6):511-6, 1993 Nov.

145. Mailer, K., et al., Age-related changes in anti-oxidative enzymes in cardiomyopathic hamster hearts, Mech of Ageing & Develop, 59(1-2):37-45, 1991 Jun 14.

146. Li, Y., et al., Correlation of selenium, glutathione peroxidase activity and lipoperoxidation rates in dilated cardiomyopathy, Chin Med J - Peking, 102(9):670-1, 1989 Sep.

147. Kennedy, T., et al., Role of reactive oxygen species in reperfusion injury of the rabbit lung, J Clin Investig, 83(4):1326-35, 1989 Apr.

148. Eichholzer, M., et al., Inverse correlation between essential antioxidants in plasma and subsequent risk to develop cancer, ischemic heart disease and stroke respectively: 12-year follow-up of the prospective Basel study, EXS, 62:398-410, 1992

149. Ringer, T., et al., Beta-carotene's effects on serum lipoproteins and immunologic indices in humans, Am J Clinical Nutri, 53(3):688-94,1991 Mar.

150. Riemersma, R., et al., Risk of angina pectoris and plasma concentrations of vitamins A, C, and E and carotene, Lancet, 337(8732):1-5, 1991 Jan 5.

151. Leibovitz, B., et al., Dietary supplements of vitamin E, beta-carotene, coenzyme Q10 and

selenium protect tissues against lipid peroxidation in rat tissue slices, J Nutri, 120(1):97-104, 1990 Jan.

152. Harris, W., The prevention of atherosclerosis with antioxidants, Clin Cardiol, 15(9):636-40, 1992 Sep.

153. Salonen, J., et al., Effects of antioxidant supplementation on platelet function: a randomized pair-matched, placebo-controlled, double-blind trial in men with low antioxidant status, Am J Clinical Nutri, 53(5):1222-9, 1991 May.

154. Mogelvang, B., Can arteriosclerosis be prevented by antioxants? Nordisk Medicin, 107(2):53-6, 1992.

155. Konovalova, G., et al., The role of free-radical inhibitors of lipid peroxidation in protecting the myocardium from ischemic damage, Arkhiv Patologii, 51(6):19-24, 1989.

156. Gey, K., et al., Plasma vitamins E and A inversely correlated to morality from ischemic heart disease in cross-cultural epidemiology, Ans N.Y. Acad of Sciences, 570:268-82, 1989.

157. Alexander, J., et al., Future prospects for adjunctive therapy: pharmacologic and nutritional approaches to immune system modulation, Critical Care Med, 18(2 Suppl):s159-64, 1990 Feb.

158. Gey, K., Plasma vitamin A and E correlate inversely with coronary mortality, 34(2)78-80, 1989.

159. Laughton, M., et al., Inhibition of mammalian 5-lipoxygenase and cyclo-oxygenase by flavonoids and phenolic dietary additives. relationship to antioxidant activity and to iron ion-reducing ability, Biochem Pharmacol, 42(9):1673-81, 1991 Oct. 9.

160. Poliukhovich, G., et al., Efficacy of various antioxidants in experimental ischemia and myocardial infarct in the rat, Voprosy Meditsinskoi Khimii, 37(4):54-6, 1991 Jul-Aug.

161. Retsky, K., et al., Ascorbic acid oxidation product(s) protect human low density lipoprotein against atherogenic modification. anti-rather than pro-oxidant activity of vitamin C in the presence of metal ions, J Bone & Min Res, 268(2):1304-9, 1993 Jan 15.

162. Trout, D., Vitamin C and cardiovascular risk factors, Am J Clinical Nutri, 53(1 Suppl):322S-325S, 1991 Jan.

163. Harris, W., The prevention of atherosclerosis with antioxidants, Clin Cardiol, 15(9):636-40, 1992 Sep.

164. Harris, W., The prevention of atherosclerosis with antioxidants, Clin Cardiol, 15(9):636-40, 1992 Sep.

165. Alexander, J., et al., Future prospects for adjunctive therapy: pharmacologic and nutritional approaches to immune system modulation, Critical Care Med, 18(2 Suppl):s159-64, 1990 Feb.

166. Janero, D., Therapeutic potential of vitamin E against myocardial ischemic-reperfusion injury, Free Rad Biol & Med, 10(5):315-24, 1991.

167. Gey, K., The antioxidant hypothesis of cardiovascular disease: epidemiology and mechanisms, Biochem Soc Transact, 18(6):1041-5, 1990 Dec.

168. Gey, K., et al., Inverse correlation between plasma vitamin e and mortality from ischemic heart disease in cross-cultural epidemiology, Am J Clinical Nutri, 53(1 Suppl):326s-334s, 1991 Jan.

169. Gey, K., et al., Plasma vitamins E and A inversely correlated to mortality from ischemic heart disease in cross-cultural epidemiology, Ans N.Y. Acad of Sciences, 570:268-82, 1989

170. Yang, Q., et al., Effect of sodium nitrite on myocardial glutathione peroxidase and protective action of vitamin E and selenium, Biomed & Environ Sci, 4(4):373-5, 1991 Dec.

171. Lui, S., et al., Damage to hepatic thyroxine 5-deiodination induced by pathogenic factors of keshan disease and the preventive effects of selenium and vitamin E, Biomed & Environ Sci, 4(4):359-65, 1991 Dec.

172. Riemersma, R., et al., Risk of angina pectoris and plasma concentrations of vitamins A, C, and E and carotene, Lancet, 337(8732):1-5, 1991 Jan 5.

173. Eichholzer, M., et al., Inverse correlation between essential antioxidants in plasma and subsequent risk to develop cancer, ischemic heart disease and stroke respectively: 12-year follow-up of the prospective Basel study, EXS, 62:398-410, 1992

174. Hendler, Dr. S., The Complete Guide to Anti-Aging Nutrients, Simon and Schuster, New York, 1985

175. DuBois, F., et al., Chromium: physiologic role and implications in human pathology, Pathologie Biologie, 39(8):801-8, 1991 Oct.

176. Yoshimoto, S., et al., Effect of chromium administration on glucose tolerance in stroke-prone spontaneously hypertensive rats with steptozotocin-induced diabetes, Metabolism:

Clin & Exper, 41(6):636-42, 1992 Jun.

177. Mossop, R., Trivalent chromium, in atherosclerosis and diabetes, Cen African J Med, 37(11):369-74, 1991.

178. Anderson, R., Chromium, glucose tolerance, and diabetes, Biol Trace Element Res, 32:19-24, 1992 Jan-Mar.

179. Aharoni, A., et al., Hair chromium content of women with gestational diabetes compared with nondiabetic pregnant women, Am J Clinical Nutri, 55(1):104-7, 1992 Jan.

180. Hendler, Dr. S., 1985, ibid, quoting a medical study published by Newman in J of Clin Chem, 24:541, 1978.

181. Hendler, Dr. S., 1985, ibid, quoting a medical study published in the Am J of Clin Nutri, 34:2670, 1981.

182. Roeback, J. Jr., et al., Effects of chromium supplementation on serum high-density lipoprotein controlled trial, Annals Internal Med, 115(12):917-24, 1991 Dec 15.

183. Abraham, A., et al., Chromium and cholesterol-induced atherosclerosis in rabbits, Annals Nutri & Metabol, 35(4):203-7, 1991.

184. Press, R., et al., The effect of chromium picolinate on serum cholesterol and apolipoprotein fractions in human subjects, West J Med, 152(1):41-5, 1990 Jan.

185. Zimmer, H., et al., Myocardial infarction in rats: effects of metabolic and pharmacologic interventions, Basic Res in Cardiolo, 84(3):332-43, 1989 May-Jun.

186. Bech, O., et al., Effects of long-term coenzyme Q10 and captopril treatment on survival and functional capacity in rats with experimentally induced heart infarction, J Pharmacol & Exper Therap, 255(1):346-50, 1990 Oct.

187. Okamoto, H., et al., Effect of coenzyme Q10 on structural alterations in the renal membrane of stroke-prone spontaneously hypertensive rats, Biochem Med & Metabolic Biol, 45(2):216-26, 1991 Apr.

188. Momomura, S., et al., Coenzyme Q10 attenuates the progression of cardiomyopathy in hamsters, Jap Heart J, 32(1):101-10, 1991 Jan.

189. Ketagiri, T., et al., Protection of acute ischemic myocardial injury by pharmacological intervention, Jap Circ J, 53(9):1108-14, 1989 Sep.

190. Kato, T., et al., Reduction in blood viscosity by treatment with coenzyme Q10 in patients with ischemic heart disease, Internat'l J Clin Phamacol, 28(3):123-6, 1990 Mar.

191. Ketagiri, T., et al., Protection of acute ischemic myocardial injury by pharmacological intervention, Jap Circ J, 53(9):1108-14, 1989 Sep.

192. Zimmer, H., et al., Myocardial infarction in rats: effects of metabolic and pharmacologic interventions, Basic Res in Cardiolo, 84(3):332-43, 1989 May-Jun.

193. Karlsson, J., et al., Ischaemic heart disease, skeletal muscle fibres and exercise capacity, Euro Heart J, 13(6):758-62, 1992 Jun.

194. Wang, Y., et al., Effect of ubiquinone on ischemic arrhythmia in conscious rats, Acta Pharmaologica Sinica, 12(3):202-6, 1991 May.

195. Wang, Y., et al., Effect of ubiquinone on ischemic arrhythmia in conscious rats, Acta Pharmaologica Sinica, 12(3):202-6, 1991 May.

196. Karlsson, J., et al., Muscle fibre types, ubiquinone content and exercise capacity in hypertension and effort angina, Ans Med, 23(3):339-44, 1991 Aug.

197. Manzoli, U., et al., Coenzyme Q10 in dilated cardiomyopathy, Lipids, 12(3):173-8, 1990.

198. Hendler, Dr. S., The Complete Guide to Anti-Aging Nutrients, p 270, Simon and Schuster, New York, 1985, quoting a medical study published in the Resident and Staff Physician, 29:102, 1983.

199. Manzoli, U., et al., Coenzyme Q10 in dilated cardiomyopathy, Lipids, 12(3):173-8, 1990.

200. Sugawara, H., et al., Inhibition of ubiquinone synthesis in isolated rat heart under an ischemic condition, Internat'l J Biochem, 22(5):477-80, 1990.

201. Matsushima, T., et al., Protection by coenzyme Q10 of canine myocardial reperfusion injury after preservation, J Thoracic & Cardiovas Surg, 103(5):945-51.

202. Lennon, John and Shealy, Dr. C. Norman, Postural and respiratory modulation of auto nomic function, pain and health, American Journal of Pain Management, 4(1): 36-39, 1994.

203. Bean, Constance, The Better Back Book, William Morrow & Company, New York, NY, 1989.

204. Henry, Linda, Fit For Motherhood, Muscle & Fitness, July 1995.

205. Noble, Elizabeth, Essential Exercises for the Childbearing Year, Houghton Mifflin Company, Boston, MA, 1988.

206. Olkin, Sylvia Klein, Positive Parenting Fitness and Positive Pregnancy Fitness, Avery Publishing, Garden City Park, NY, 1992, 1987.

207. Jackson, Ian, The Breathplay Approach to Whole Life Fitness, Doubleday & Company, New York, NY, 1986 and Speads, Carola H., Breathing: The ABC's, Harper Colophon Books, New York, NY, 1978.

BIBLIOGRAPHY

Antonello, Jean, *How to Become Naturally Thin by Eating More*, Avon Books, New York, NY, 1989.

Appenzeller, Otto M.D., *Sports Medicine, Fitness, Training and Injuries, 3rd edition*, Urban and Schwartzberg, Munich, Germany, 1988.

Bailey, Covert, *Smart Exercise*, Houghton Mifflin Company, Boston, MA, 1994.

Balch, Dr. James F., M.D. and Balch, Phyllis, *Prescription for Nutritional Healing*, Avery Publishing, Garden City Park, NY, 1990.

Basmajian, Dr. John, *The Human Body: Muscles, The Magic of Motion*, Torstar Books, New York, NY, 1985.

Bean, Constance, *The Better Back Book*, William Morrow, New York, NY, 1989.

Bragg, Paul, *The Natural Way to Reduce*, Health Science Publishers, Santa Barbara, CA, 1984.

Bricklin, Mark, *Lose Weight Naturally*, Rodale Press, Emmaus, PA, 1989.

Brody, Jane, *Jane Brody's Nutrition Book*, W.W. Norton & Company, New York, NY, 1981.

Concoby, Robert, *Discovered: Nature's Secret Fountains of Youth*, Hanford Press, Canton, OH, 1993.

Craig, Jenny, *What Have You Got to Lose*, Villard Books, New York, NY, 1992.

Darden, Ellington, Ph.D., *High-Intensity Strength Training*, Putnam Publishing Company, New York, NY, 1992.

Feldenkrais, Moshe, *The Potent Self*, Harper and Row, San Francisco, CA, 1985.

Franks, B. Don and Howley, Edward T., *Fitness Facts: The Healthy Living Handbook*, Human Kinetics Books, Champaign, IL, 1989.

Good Food and Fitness, Better Homes and Garden Books, Des Moines, IA, 1981.

Gutfeld, Greg, *Banish your Potbelly: A Man's Guide to Fighting Fat*, Rodale Press, Emmaus, PA, 1993.

Hay, James and Reid, J.Gavin, *The Anatomical and Mechanical Bases of Human Motion*, Prentice-Hall, Englewood Cliffs, New Jersey, 1982.

Jackson, Ian, *The Breathplay Approach to Whole Life Fitness*, Doubleday & Company, New York, NY, 1986.

Katahn, Martin, *Beyond Diet*, W.W. Norton & Company, New York, NY, 1984.

Lennon, John and Shealy, Dr. C. Norman, *"Postural and Respiratory Modulation of Autonomic Function, Pain and Health,"* American Journal of Pain Management, Volume 4, Number 1, January, 1994

Logue, A.W., *The Psychology of Eating and Drinking*, W. H. Freeman & Company, New York, NY, 1986.

Mayer, Jean, *A Diet for Living*, David McKay Company, New York, NY, 1975.

McDougall, Dr. John A., M.D., *The McDougall Program for Maximum Weight Loss*, Penguin Books, New York, NY, 1994.

Netzer, Corinne, *The Complete Book of Food Counts*, Dell Publishing, 1994.

Noble, Elizabeth, *Essential Exercises for the Childbearing Year*, Houghton Mifflin Company, Boston, MA, 1988.

Olkin, Sylvia Klein, *Positive Parenting Fitness*, Avery Publishing, Garden City Park, NY, 1992.

Olkin, Sylvia Klein, *Positive Pregnancy Fitness*, Avery Publishing, Garden City Park, NY, 1987.

Ornish, Dr. Dean, M.D., *Eat More, Weigh Less*, Harper Collins, New York, NY, 1993.

Patton, Kevin and Thibodeau, Gary, *Anatomy and Physiology, 2nd edition*, Mosby-Year Books, St. Louis, MO, 1993.

Pennington, Jean A.T., *Bowes and Church's Food Values of Portions Commonly Used* 16th ed., J.B. Lippincott Company, Philadelphia, PA, 1994.

Speads, Carola H., *Breathing: The ABC's*, Harper Colophon Books, New York, NY, 1978.

Stare, Frederick J., and Whelan, Elizabeth M., *Eat OK-Feel OK*, North Quincy, MA Christopher Co., 1978.

Stare, Frederick J., and McWilliams, Margaret, *Living Nutrition*, 3rd ed., John Wiley & Sons, New York, NY, 1981.

Todd, Mabel Ellsworth, *The Thinking Body*, Dance Horizons, New York, NY, 1937.

Tver, David F. and Russell, Percy, Ph.D., *The Nutrition and Health Encyclopedia* Van Nostrand Reinhold Company, New York, NY, 1981.